Drugs and Protocols Common to Prehospital and Emergency Care

The Jones and Bartlett Pocket-Sized Nursing Reference Series

Chemotherapy Care Plans: Designs for Nursing Care
Barton Burke/Wilkes/Ingwersen

Drugs and Protocols Common to Prehospital and Emergency Care
Cummings

The EMS Pocket Drug Manual: A Quick Reference Guide to Over 3,500 Drugs
Dillman

1991-1992 Handbook of Intravenous Medications
Nentwich

Handbook of Oncology Nursing, Second Edition
Johnson/Gross

Memory Bank for Chemotherapy, Second Edition
Preston/Wilfinger

Memory Bank for Critical Care: EKGs and Cardiac Drugs, Third Edition
Ervin

Memory Bank for Hemodynamic Monitoring The Pulmonary Artery Catheter, Second Edition
Ervin/Long

Memory Bank for Intravenous Therapy Second Edition
Weinstein

Memory Bank for Medications, Second Edition
Kostin/Sieloff

Oncology Nursing Drug Handbook
Wilkes/Ingwersen/Barton Burke

Ready Reference for Critical Care
Strawn/Stewart

Drugs and Protocols Common to Prehospital and Emergency Care

P. Howard Cummings, EdD, RN
Associate Professor
The University of North Carolina
at Wilmington

Jones and Bartlett Publishers
Boston *London*

Editorial, Sales, and Customer Service Offices

Jones and Bartlett Publishers
One Exeter Plaza
Boston, MA 02116

Jones and Bartlett Publishers International
PO Box 1498
London W6 7RS England

Library of Congress Cataloging-in-Publication Data

Cummings, P. Howard.
Drugs and protocols common to prehospital and emergency care / P. Howard Cummings.
p. cm.
Includes bibliographical references and index.
ISBN 0-86720-214-9
1. Drugs—Handbooks, manuals, etc. 2. Emergency medicine—Handbooks, manuals, etc. 3. Emergency medical technicians—Handbooks, manuals, etc. 4. Emergency nursing—Handbooks, manuals, etc. I. Title.
[DNLM: 1. Drug therapy—handbooks. 2. Emergencies—handbooks. WB 39 C971d}
RM301.12.C85 1993
615.5'8—dc20
DNLM/DLC
for Library of Congress 93-49472
CIP

Printed in the United States of America
97 96 95 94 93 10 9 8 7 6 5 4 3 2 1

Dedication

To the volunteers of Seneca Rescue Squad, Seneca, South Carolina, who are devoted, unselfish and loving Samaritans for whom I care very much

and

To my best friend, Craig Steven Nine, whose unconditional friendship has been and continues to be very special to me. Always remember the commitments that are MOST important: your family, your career (EMS or otherwise), and your "best friend for life"!

P.H.C. (612)

Contributors

Sally P. Cummings, EdD, RN
Assistant Professor
The University of North Carolina
at Wilmington

Anita Hyler, BSN, RN, (MS in Nursing candidate)
Staff Nurse—Critical Care
Oconee Memorial Hospital
Seneca, South Carolina

Carolyn Mega, BSN, RN, (MS in Nursing candidate)
Staff Nurse—Greenville Hospital System
Neonatal Intensive Care
Greenville, South Carolina

Contents

Preface

This book is designed to assist health care workers to be able to obtain vital information concerning the preparation and administration of drugs and to have quick access to protocols commonly used in prehospital and emergency situations. It is primarily a pharmacological reference for those persons faced with administering drugs without sufficient time or resources to research the drugs' class, uses, action, usual dosage and route for adults and children, rapid and gradual adverse/side effects, contraindications, special precautions, other special information, and antidotes for severe and other reactions. It also offers vital information relative to protocols, scales, formulas, scores, indexes, and tables presented in a simple format that can be read in a very short time.

This book is not meant to contain all there is to know about the pharmacological agents included, but it offers what the author views as essential information to know before administration.

The primary audience is health personnel (physicians, nurses, paramedics, students) in prehospital and emergency settings. But personnel in critical care and general medical-surgical areas can benefit from this book as well. The book's compactness is purposeful—to allow it to fit into drug boxes and the pockets of lab jackets and health uniforms.

The drug monographs appear in alphabetical order according to the drugs' generic name (in capital letters). Because many drugs have numerous registered trade names, the author chose to list only simple trade names for each drug category. This does not indicate bias, preference, or endorsement.

Part One includes a CPR ready reference guide, in addition to tables for drugs commonly used during cardiac arrest. There is an adult and pediatric table that lists the drugs, their uses, actions, dosage/route, and dosage forms in a simple and easy-to-read format that facilitates drug administration during a code situation. A drug calculation table for pediatric drugs is included to facilitate their quick use in a code situation. Advanced Cardiac Life Support algorithms for ventricular fibrillation, asystole, electromechanical dissociation, ventricular tachycardia, and bradycardia are also included.

Part Two includes a table of common intravenous solutions. The solutions are categorized as saline, dextrose, combination saline and dextrose, plasma, and serum solutions. Electrolyte and calorie content for each intravenous fluid are offered, with each classified according to its osmolarity, uses, action, and relative contraindications.

Part Three consists of monographs of more than 150 drugs considered common or frequently used in prehospital and emergency settings. Each monograph contains brief statements about the drug's class, uses, and action. It then lists usual adult and pediatric doses, as well as the available routes of administration. An effort has been made to use common dosages and conversions to facilitate computing and validating dosages. Still, dosages may need to be evaluated according to each patient's needs and situation at the time of administration. Each monograph lists common adverse/side effects that might be rapid, and those considered gradual, as well as contraindications, special precautions, and other special information needed by the person administering the drug. The last section of each monograph lists antidotes for rapid as well as other reactions from the drugs, including drugs that might be used to counteract a hypersensitivity reaction whenever possible.

Part Four includes conversion tables and formulas for various dosage forms to assist the user in making calculations and conversions swiftly and efficiently. Whenever possible, the author advises the use of body surface area (M^2) in dosing children, because this method is the most accurate form of drug dosing in children, as well as unusually slim or obese adults. Conversion tables for metric-to-apothecary, pounds-to-kilograms, and inches-to-centimeters are included, as well as formulas for calculating intravenous drip rates.

Part Five includes a variety of adult and pediatric scales, indexes, and scores that are commonly used in defining the severity of injury of a victim. Included are Glasgow coma scales, prehospital index, trauma scores, burn charts and tables, infant Apgar score, pediatric normal vital sign parameters, and an electrocardiogram interpretation guide.

The Appendix includes a list of common abbreviations and a resource bibliography. The blank drug monographs may be used to list additional drugs not covered in this book.

While using this text, if you discover inconsistencies in what you consider usual drug information, or if you feel that certain drugs ought to be added or omitted from future editions, please contact the author through the publisher. The author hopes that this book meets a long-identified need and that those who will ultimately benefit most from this book are the patients who require quality care and treatment.

Acknowledgments

I wish to express my deep appreciation to the contributors for sharing their knowledge and expertise in nursing and medicine for the preparation of this text. Their sustained input, involvement, and encouragement made the completion of this reference a reality of a dream.

I would also like to thank all my students in adult nursing at Clemson University, Clemson, South Carolina, as well as my First Responder, EMT and paramedic friends and colleagues for their interest, encouragement, and support. It was their communication of the need for such a reference that encouraged me to continue my research and writing so that they could use the book in their growth toward professionalism and accountability in their chosen health professions.

I am deeply grateful to my typist, Nancy Carls, who spent many hours of her time—over and above her usual duties—to type and proofread the manuscript. Most of all, I am forever indebted to my family: Sally, Amanda, and Joshua, for their patience, support, and tolerance when deadlines were near.

Part One
Cardiac Arrest Tables

CPR Ready Reference

Parameter	Adults	Children	Infants
Rescue breathing: If the victim has a pulse, give 1 breath every	5 sec	4 sec	3 sec
Hand position for compression	Trace ribs to notch, 2 fingers above xyphoid process	Same as adult	1 finger width below nipple line
Compression type	2 hands stacked with heel of 1 hand on sternum	Heel of 1 hand on sternum	2 (or 3) fingers on sternum
Rate of compressions	80–100/min	80–100/min	At least 100/min
Depth of compressions	1½–2 inches	1–1½ inches	½–1 inch
Compression/ ventilation ratio	1 rescuer, 15:2 2 rescuers, 5:1	1 rescuer, 5:1	1 rescuer, 5:1

*Conscious choking victim	6–10 abdominal thrusts; reassess airway	6–10 abdominal thrusts; reassess airway	4 back blows; 4 chest thrusts; reassess airway
*Unconscious choking victim	6–10 abdominal thrusts; finger sweep; reattempt ventilations	6–10 abdominal thrusts; look for foreign object; reattempt ventilations	4 back blows, 4 chest thrusts, look for foreign object & reattempt ventilations

*Changes anticipated based on October 28, 1992 publication of *JAMA* (vol. 268, no. 16).

Adult Cardiac Resuscitation Drug Table

Drug	Uses	Action	Usual Dosage/ Route	Dosage Forms
LIDOCAINE HYDROCHLORIDE (Xylocaine HCL)	*Cardiac dysrhythmias (6 or more PVCs/min, during cardiac arrest & R on T phenomena *Prophylactically after a myocardial infarction to prevent primary ventricular fibrillation	*Suppresses dysrhythmias of ventricular origin by decreasing myocardial automaticity *Terminates gating function of Purkinje fibers *Increases fibrillation threshold	50–100 mg (approx. 1 mg/kg) IV bolus and may be repeated every 3–5 min as needed to max dose of 300 mg followed by continuous IV infusion of 20–50 mcg/kg/min (1–4 mg/min in 70-kg patient) to establish blood levels of 1.4–6.0 mcg/ml *To prevent recurrent ventricular fibrillation continue for at least 24 hr after	**Prefilled syringes:** 50 mg/5 ml (1%); 100 mg/10 ml (2%); 100 mg/5 ml (1%); 1 gm/25 ml (4%); 1 gm/50 ml (2%); **Vials:** 50 ml (20 mg/ml); **Ampules:** 5 ml (20 mg/ml)

			IV Mixture: 1 gm/500 ml D_5W = 2 mg/ml; 1 gm/250 ml D_5W = 4 mg/ml	
ADENOSINE (Adenocard)	*Paroxysmal superventricular tachycardia (PSVT)	*Slows AV node conduction by interrupting re-entry pathways to the AV node	*IV bolus 6 mg; if no response after 1–2 min, give 12 mg rapid IV bolus; may repeat 12 mg IV bolus × 1	**Ampules:** 3 mg/ml
EPINEPHRINE (Adrenalin Chloride)	*Poor cardiac compression & rhythm *Ventricular fibrillation and asystole	*Increases heart rate *Increases myocardial contractile force *Increases systemic vascular resistance *Increases arterial blood pressure	0.5–1.0 mg IV, SL, or endotracheal tube followed by 0.5 mg at 5-min intervals (5 ml of a 1:10,000 solution)	**Prefilled syringes:** 10 ml (1.0 mg in 1:10,000 dilution) **Ampules:** 1 ml (1.0 mg in 1:1,000 dilution)

(cont'd.)

Adult Cardiac Resuscitation Drug Table (cont'd.)

Drug	Uses	Action	Usual Dosage/ Route	Dosage Forms
EPINEPHRINE (Adrenalin Chloride) (cont'd.)		*Increases myocardial oxygen consumption *Increases automaticity *Converts fine ventricular fibrillation to coarse ventricular fibrillation once acidosis corrected *Increased coronary and cerebral blood flow		
ATROPINE SULFATE	*Frequent ventricular ectopic beats *Severe bradycardia with	*Reduces vagal tone and accelerates rate of discharge of the SA node	1 mg IV followed by 0.5 mg IV at 5-min intervals not exceeding total dose of 2.0 mg	**Prefilled syringes:** 10 mg/10 ml **Syringes:** 0.5 mg/5 ml

	hypotension *High degree AV block *Slow ventricular rates	*Improves AV conduction		**Vials:** 0.4 mg/ml or 0.5 mg/ml
PROCAINAMIDE (Pronestyl, Procamide, Procapan)	*Ventricular extrasystole *Recurrent ventricular tachycardia not controlled by LIDOCAINE *To convert supraventricular arrhythmias	*Depresses excitability of cardiac muscle and slows conduction to the atrium, bundle of HIS, and ventricular muscle	100 mg over 2–5 min and repeat every 5 min up to 1 gram or follow bolus done with constant infusion at 2–6 mg/min	**Vials:** 1 gm/10 ml; 1 gm/2 ml
BRETYLIUM TOSYLATE (Bretylol)	*Ventricular antidysrhythmic *Increase ventricular threshold *Ventricular tachycardia refractory to LIDOCAINE	*Suppresses ventricular fibrillation within mins and ventricular dysrhythmias over approx. 20 min	5 mg/kg undiluted rapid IV push, and repeated as needed. May increase dose to 10 mg/kg if ventricular fibrilla-	**Ampules:** 500 mg/10 ml

(cont'd.)

Adult Cardiac Resuscitation Drug Table (cont'd.)

Drug	Uses	Action	Usual Dosage/ Route	Dosage Forms
BRETYLIUM TOSYLATE (Bretylol) (cont'd.)			tion persists & repeated at 15-to-30 min intervals; max dose 30 mg/kg	
VERAPAMIL (Calan)	*To treat paroxysmal supraventricular tachycardia not requiring cardioversion	*Reduces myocardial oxygen consumption *Reduces systemic vascular resistance *Coronary vasodilation *Slows conduction & prolongs refractoriness in the AV node	0.075–0.15 mg/kg IV over 1 min then 0.15 mg/kg 30 min after first dose; max 10 mg	**Vials:** 2.5 mg/ml

SODIUM BICARBONATE ($NaHCO_3$)	*Metabolic acidosis	*Increases electrical threshold and spontaneous activity of the heart *Increases ventricular contractile force *Increases cardiac responsiveness to catecholamines (EPINEPHRINE)	1 mEq/kg IV initially & may be repeated × 1, then 0.5 mEq/kg every 10 min thereafter until pH and base deficits are determined **Formula:** Dosage in ml of 1.5% solution = (60) − (plasma CO_2) × 0.8 body weight in lbs	**Prefilled syringes:** 50 mEq/50 ml **Ampules:** 44.6 mEq/50 ml **Bottles:** 297.5 mEq/500 ml
DOPAMINE (Intropin)	*Cardiogenic shock *Low BP	*Increases cardiac, renal, mesenteric output in small doses (1–2 mcg/kg/min) *Increases cardiac output in moderate doses (2–10	2–10 mcg/kg/min and increased until BP and urine output responds; max dose 20–50 mcg/kg/min; Infusion rate should be adjusted to	**Ampules:** 200 mg/5 ml **IV Mixture:** 200 mg/250 mg D_5W or D_5LR = 800 mcg/ml;

(cont'd.)

Drug	Uses	Action	Usual Dosage/ Route	Dosage Forms
DOPAMINE (Intropin) (cont'd.)		mcg/kg/min) *Causes peripheral vasoconstriction, increasing BP and heart rate in large doses (10 mcg/kg/min) *Constricts renal and mesenteric vessels to diminish blood flow in very large doses (> 20 mcg/kg/min) *Increases systemic vascular resistance	maintain desired effect without decreasing urine output	200 mg/500 ml D_5W or D_5LR = 400 mcg/ml
ISOPROTERENOL (Isuprel)	*Bradycardia due to heart block	*Beta-adrenergic receptor stimula-	5–10 mcg/kg IV followed by an IV	**Vials:** 1 mg

	*Sinus bradycardia if ATROPINE SULFATE is unsuccessful *Cardiac standstill *Ventricular dysrhythmias due to AV nodal block	tor *Increases cardiac output *Increases myocardial oxygen demand *Increases venous return to the heart *Decreases peripheral vascular resistance *Increases BP due to increase in cardiac output	infusion at a rate of 0.1 mcg/kg/min titrated according to heart rate & rhythm response not to exceed 1.5 mcg/kg/min	**IV Mixture:** 1 mg/500 ml D_5W = 2 mcg/ml; 1 mg/250 ml D_5W = 4 mcg/ml
CALCIUM CHLORIDE, CALCIUM GLUCONATE, CALCIUM GLUCEPTATE	*Ventricular standstill *Profound cardiovascular collapse (electromechanical dissociation)	*Increases myocardial contractile force *Enhances ventricular excitability	CALCIUM CHLORIDE: 2.5–5 ml of 10% solution (.25–.5 gm) repeated at 10-min intervals (3.4–6.8 mEq Ca^{++}) CALCIUM GLUCONATE: 10 ml	**Prefilled syringes:** 10 ml CALCIUM CHLORIDE 10% (1 gm); 5 ml CALCIUM

(cont'd.)

Drug	Uses	Action	Usual Dosage/ Route	Dosage Forms
CALCIUM CHLORIDE, CALCIUM GLUCONATE, CALCIUM GLUCEPTATE (cont'd.)			of 10% solution (1 gm) repeated at 10-min intervals (4.8 mEq Ca^{++}) CALCIUM GLUCEPTATE: 5 ml (1.1 gm) repeated at 10-min intervals (4.5 mEq Ca^{++})	GLUCEPTATE (1.1 gm); 10 ml CALCIUM GLUCONATE 10%
PROPRANOLOL HCL (Inderal)	*Ventricular tachycardia *Recurrent ventricular fibrillation *Tachydysrhythmias due to digitalis toxicity	*Beta-adrenergic receptor blocker *Interferes with adrenergic bronchodilator activity and can cause bronchospasm *Antidysrhythmic when LIDOCAINE is not effective	1–3 mg IV slowly (1 mg/min) repeated as needed to a max dose of 3–5 mg	Vials: 1 mg/1 ml diluted in 10 ml D_5W

Pediatric Cardiac Resuscitation Drug Table

Drug	Uses	Action	Usual Dosage/ Route (See Calculation Table)	Dosage Forms
EPINEPHRINE	*Bradydysrhythmias *Asystole *Asthma *Anaphylaxis	*Cardiovascular & vasopressor action *Increases heart rate, cardiac output, myocardial oxygen consumption & force of contraction *Bronchodilator	*0.01 mg/kg of 1:10,000 solution (0.1 ml/kg) IV or IO every 5 min. ET dose 0.1 mg/kg of 1:1,000 solution diluted and administered via catheter every 5 min.	**Prefilled syringes:** 10 ml (1 mg in 1:10,000 dilution). **Ampules:** 1 ml (1 mg in 1:1,000 dilution). Must be diluted in 10 ml NS.

(cont'd.)

Pediatric Cardiac Resuscitation Drug Table (cont'd.)

Drug	Uses	Action	Usual Dosage/ Route (See Calculation Table)	Dosage Forms
ATROPINE SULFATE	*Symptomatic bradycardia *Ventricular asystole	*Antidysrhythmic action improves AV conduction; *Reduces vagal tone	*IV, ET: 0.02 mg/kg; may repeat every 5 min up to 1 mg for children; *Minimum dose is 0.1 mg to prevent paradoxical bradycardia	0.5 mg/5ml syringe
SODIUM BICARBONATE ($NaHCO_3$)	*Prolonged cardiac arrest *Documented metabolic acidosis	*Increases cardiac response to EPINEPHRINE; *Alkalizing buffering action	*IV: 1mEq/kg dilute with equal amounts of D_5W; may repeat every 10 min for a max of 50 mEq	8.4% sol (1 mEq/ml)
CALCIUM CHLORIDE	*Prolonged cardiac standstill with hypocal-	*Increases myocardial contractile force	*IV: 20 mg/kg; given slow IV 1 ml/min; may re-	10% sol (100 mg/ml)

	cemia clearly present	*Enhances ventricular excitability	peat in 10 min	
LIDOCAINE	*Ventricular fibrillation	*Suppresses ventricular dysrhythmias	*IV, ET: 1 mg/kg; may repeat every 5–10 min up to 3 times	20 mg/ml ABBOJECT
ISOPROTERENOL (Isuprel)	*Bradycardia due to heart block *Sinus bradycardia if ATROPHINE SULFATE is unsuccessful *Cardiac standstill	*Beta-adrenergic receptor stimulator *Increases cardiac output *Increases myocardial oxygen demand *Increases venous return to the heart *Decreases peripheral vascular resistance *Increases BP due to increase in cardiac output	*IV: 0.1–1.0 mcg/kg/min titrated according to heart rate & rhythm response	**Vials:** 1 mg **IV mixture:** 1 mg/500 ml D_5W = 2 mcg/ml; 1 mg/250 ml D_5W = 4 mcg/ml

(cont'd.)

Pediatric Cardiac Resuscitation Drug Table (cont'd.)

Drug	Uses	Action	Usual Dosage/ Route (See Calculation Table)	Dosage Forms
NALOXONE (Narcan)	*Opioid-induced respiratory depression	*Antagonist to most of opioid effects	*IV, IM, ET: 0.01 mg/kg; may repeat every 2–3 min up to 0.1 mg/kg total dose	0.02 mg/ml 0.04 mg/ml dilute to make 0.02 mg/ml sol
DOPAMINE (Intropin)	*Shock *Hypotension or poor peripheral perfusion	*Vasopressor action *Vasodilation in renal, mesenteric, coronary, & intracerebral vascular beds *Cardiac stimulant in low-to-moderate doses *Renal vasoconstriction and increased periph-	*IV infusion of 5–10 mcg/kg/min; increase to max of 20 mcg/kg/min	200 mg/5ml amp; mix 200 mg/250 ml D_5W

		eral resistance in high doses		
DIAZEPAM (Valium)	*Seizures *Tetanic muscle spasms	*Depresses CNS *Suppresses spread of seizure activity in cortex	*IV: 0.25mg/kg slow IV bolus at rate not to exceed 5mg/min; may repeat every 15 min up to 2 times; *Max dose for children is 15 mg *Max dose for infants is 5 mg	5 mg/ml amp
AMINOPHYLLINE	*Bronchial asthma *Bronchospasm *Respiratory and myocardial stimulant in apnea	*Relaxes smooth muscle of the respiratory system	*IV: 5 mg/kg (neonates 1 mg/kg) slowly for a period of 20–30 mins 1.0 loading dose; then 0.6 mg/kg/hr continuous drip not to exceed a rate of 25 mg/min	250, 500 mg/amps; dilute in D_5W, NaCL, $D_5$1/2NS, LR or other common IV fluids

Pediatric Cardiac Resuscitation Drug Calculations
(All of the numbers in the table are reported in milliliters.)

Weight (kg) Approx. age	3 Newborn	6 3 mo	7.5 6 mo	10 1 yr	12 2 yr	14 3 yr	18 5 yr	25 8 yr	30 10 yr
EPINEPHRINE: 0.01 mg/kg 1:10,000 0.1 mg/ml (0.1 ml/kg)	0.3	0.6	0.7	1.0	1.2	1.4	1.8	2.5	3.0
ATROPINE: 0.02 mg/kg 0.1 mg/ml (0.2 ml/kg)	1.0*	1.2	1.5	2.0	2.4	2.8	3.6	5.0	6.0
NA BICARBONATE: 1 mEq/kg 1 mEq/ml (8.4% sol); dilute with equal amts of D_5W	3.0	6.0	7.5	10.0	12.0	14.0	18.0	25.0	30.0

**Note*: The minimum dose is 0.1 mg or 1.0 ml to prevent paradoxical bradycardia.

CALCIUM CHLORIDE: 20 mg/kg 100 mg/ml (10%) (0.2 ml/kg)	0.6	1.2	1.5	2.0	2.4	2.8	3.6	5.0	6.0
LIDOCAINE: 1 mg/kg 20 mg/ml (0.05 ml/kg)	0.15	0.3	0.375	0.5	0.6	0.7	0.9	1.25	1.5
ISOPROTERENOL: 0.1–1.0 mcg/kg/min (0.5 mcg/kg/min) 1 mg/500 ml D_5W (2 mcg/ml)	0.75	1.5	1.875	2.5	3.0	3.5	4.5	6.25	7.5
NALOXONE: 0.01 mg/kg 0.02 mg/ml (0.5 ml/kg) 0.4 mg/ml (0.025 ml/kg)	1.5 —	3.0 0.15	3.75 0.18	5.0 0.25	6.0 0.3	7.0 0.35	— 0.45	— 0.6	— 0.75

(cont'd.)

Pediatric Cardiac Resuscitation Drug Calculations (cont'd.)

Weight (kg) Approx. age	3 Newborn	6 3 mo	7.5 6 mo	10 1 yr	12 2 yr	14 3 yr	18 5 yr	25 8 yr	30 10 yr
DOPAMINE: 5–10 mcg/kg/min; 200 mg/5 ml; amt in ml to add to 100 cc volume for IV. Run at 1 cc/hr	2.25 to 4.5	4.5 to 9.0	5.6 to 11.2	7.5 to 15.0	9.0 to 18.0	10.5 to 21.0	13.5 to 27.0	18.7 to 37.5	22.5 to 45.0
DIAZEPAM: 0.25 mg/kg 5 mg/ml	0.15	0.3	0.37	0.5	0.6	0.7	0.9	1.25	1.5
AMINOPHYLLINE: 0.6–1 mg/kg (1 mg/kg) 250 mg/250 ml (1 mg/ml)	3.0	6.0	7.5	10.0	12.0	14.0	18.0	25.0	30.0

Volume Expanders: 15 ml/kg ALBUMIN 5% PLASMANATE 5% 0.9% NORMAL SALINE	45	90	112.5	150	180	210	270	375	450

Ventricular Fibrillation (VF) and Pulseless Ventricular Tachycardia (VT) A.C.L.S. Algorithm

Witnessed Arrest	Unwitnessed Arrest
↓	↓
Check pulse; if no pulse	Check pulse; if no pulse
↓	
Precordial thump	
↓	
Check pulse; if no pulse	

↓

CPR until a defibrillator is available

↓

Check monitor for rhythm; if VF or VT

↓

Defibrillate, 200 Joules

↓

Defibrillate, 200–300 Joules

↓

Defibrillate with up to 360 Joules

↓

CPR if no pulse

↓

Establish IV access

↓

EPINEPHRINE, 1:10,000, 0.5–1.0 mg IV push
(repeat every 5 min)

↓

Intubate if possible

↓

Defibrillate with up to 360 Joules

↓

LIDOCAINE, 1 mg/kg IV push

↓

Defibrillate with up to 360 Joules

↓

BRETYLIUM, 5 mg/kg IV push
(or LIDOCAINE 0.5 mg/kg every 8 min up to 3 mg/kg)

↓

(Consider BICARBONATE at 1 mEq/kg;
repeat ½ dose every 10 min)

↓

Defibrillate with up to 360 Joules

↓

BRETYLIUM, 10 mg/kg IV push (or LIDOCAINE as above)

↓

Defibrillate with up to 360 Joules

↓

Repeat LIDOCAINE or BRETYLIUM

↓

Defibrillate with up to 360 Joules

Asystole (Cardiac Standstill) A.C.L.S. Algorithm

If rhythm is unclear and ventricular fibrillation possible,
defibrillate as for VF if asystole is present

↓

Continue CPR

↓

Establish IV access

↓

EPINEPHRINE, 1:10,000, 0.5–1.0 mg IV push
(repeated every 5 min)

↓

Intubate when possible

↓

ATROPINE, 1.0 mg IV push (repeated in 5 min)

↓

(Consider BICARBONATE at 1 mEq/kg;
repeat ½ dose every 10 min)

↓

Consider pacing

Electromechanical Dissociation A.C.L.S. Algorithm

Continue CPR

↓

Establish IV access

↓

EPINEPHRINE, 1:10,000, 0.5–1.0 mg IV push
(repeat every 5 min)

↓

Intubate when possible

↓

(Consider BICARBONATE at 1 mEq/kg;
repeat ½ dose every 10 min)

↓

Consider hypovolemia,
Cardiac tamponate,
Tension pneumothorax,
Hypoxemia,
Acidosis,
Pulmonary embolism

Sustained Ventricular Tachycardia A.C.L.S. Algorithm

No Pulse ⟷ **Pulse Present**

Treat as VF

Stable

↓

O_2

↓

IV access

↓

LIDOCAINE, 1 mg/kg

↓

LIDOCAINE, 0.5 mg/kg every 8 min until VT resolves, or up to 3 mg/kg

↓

PROCAINAMIDE, 20 mg/min until VT resolves, or up to 1,000 mg

↓

Cardiovert as in unstable patients (consider sedation)

Unstable (chest pain dyspnea, BP, CHF, ischemia, MI)

↓

O_2

↓

IV access

↓

(Consider sedation)

↓

Cardiovert 50 Joules (may consider precordial thump first if no S & S of decreased BP, pulmonary embolus, unconsciousness)

↓

Cardiovert 100 Joules

↓

Cardiovert 200 Joules

↓

Cardiovert with up to 360 Joules

↓

If recurrent, add LIDOCAINE and cardiovert again starting at energy level previously successful; then PROCAINAMIDE or BRETYLIUM IV infusion

Bradycardia A.C.L.S. Algorithm

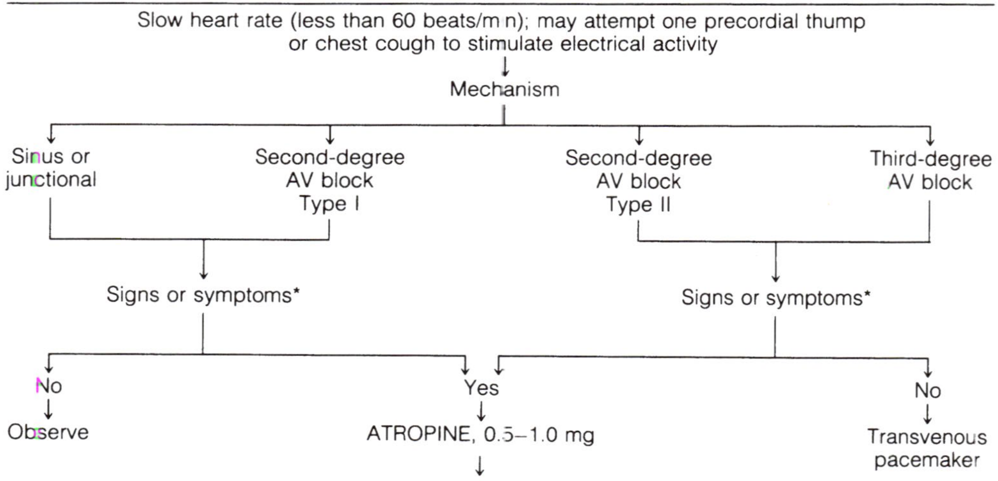

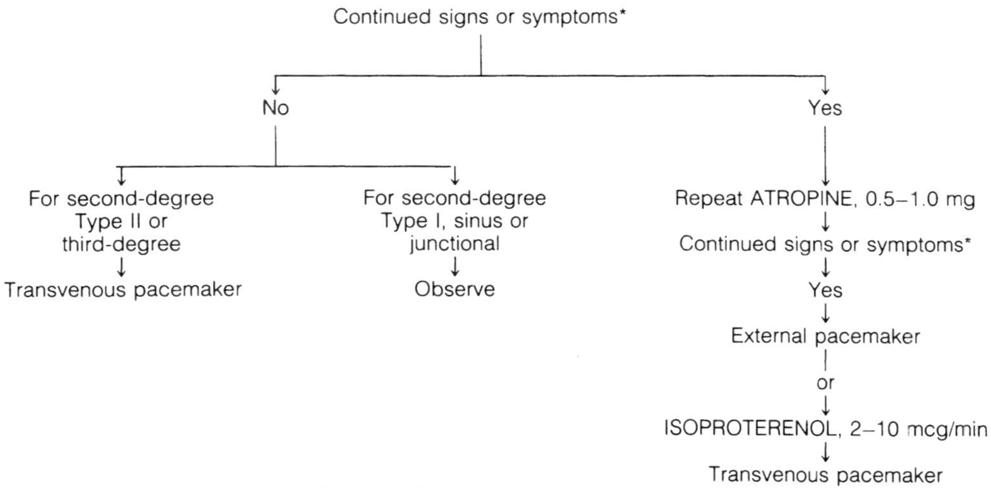

*Signs and symptoms = hypotension (SBP < 90 mmHg), PVCs, altered mental status, chest pain, dyspnea, ischemia, infarction

Paroxysmal Supraventricular Tachycardia A.C.L.S. Algorithm

PSVT

Unstable

↓

Synchronous cardioversion 75–100 Joules

↓

Synchronous cardioversion 200 Joules

↓

Synchronous cardioversion 360 Joules

↓

Correct underlying abnormalities

↓

Pharmacological therapy + cardioversion

Stable

↓

Vagal maneuvers

↓

Verapamil, 5 mg IV

↓

Verapamil, 10 mg IV (in 15–20 min)

↓

Cardioversion, DIGOXIN, β-blockers, pacing as indicated

If conversion occurs but PSVT recurs, repeated electrical cardioversion is *not* indicated. Sedation should be used as time permits.

Suppression of Ventricular Ectopy A.C.L.S. Algorithm

Assess for need for
acute suppressive therapy

↓

→ Rule out treatable cause
→ Consider serum potassium
→ Consider digitalis level
→ Consider bradycardia
→ Consider drugs

↓

LIDOCAINE, 1 mg/kg

↓

If not suppressed,
repeat LIDOCAINE, 0.5 mg/kg every 2–10 min
until no ectopy, or up to 3 mg/kg given

↓

If not suppressed,
PROCAINAMIDE 20 mg/min
until no ectopy, or up to 1,000 mg given

↓

If not suppressed,
and not contraindicated,

↓

(cont'd.)

Suppression of Ventricular Ectopy A.C.L.S. Algorithm (cont'd.)

BRETYLIUM, 5–10 mg/kg over 8–10 min

↓

If not suppressed,
consider overdrive pacing

Once ectopy resolved, maintain as follows:

- After LIDOCAINE, 1 mg/kg . . . LIDOCAINE drip, 2 mg/min
- After LIDOCAINE, 1–2 mg/kg . . . LIDOCAINE drip, 3 mg/min
- After LIDOCAINE, 2–3 mg/kg . . . LIDOCAINE drip, 4 mg/min
- After PROCAINAMIDE . . . PROCAINAMIDE drip, 1–4 mg/min (check blood level)
- After BRETYLIUM . . . BRETYLIUM drip, 2 mg/min

Part Two
Intravenous Solutions

Intravenous Solutions

Intravenous Solution	Uses	Action and Fate	Relative Contraindications
SALINE SOLUTIONS (per liter)			
–0.9 NaCl (isotonic) (154 mEq Na^+, 154 mEq Cl) –0.45 NaCl (hypotonic) (77 mEq Na^+, 77 mEq Cl) –0.2 NaCl (hypotonic) (38 mEq Na^+, 38 mEq Cl) –Lactated Ringer's (isotonic) (130 mEq Na^+, 109 mEq Cl, 4 mEq K^+, 3 mEq Ca^{++}, 28 mEq HCO_3)	To restore blood volume in hemorrhage and blood pressure in shock For fluid loss from burns, dehydration, and many similar conditions of hypovolemia For administration of intravenous medications	Given to maintain and restore electrolyte balance (the type used depends on the needs of the patient) Isotonic NaCl is used for patients with sodium depletion	CHF Circulatory insufficiency Kidney dysfunction Hypoproteinemia Hypernatremia

DEXTROSE SOLUTIONS (per liter) –5% dextrose in water (isotonic) (170 calories) –10% dextrose in water (isotonic) (340 calories) –20% dextrose in water (hypertonic) (680 calories) –50% dextrose in water (hypertonic) (1,700 calories)	For same conditions as saline solutions with added nutrients (calories) Higher concentrated solutions act as osmotic diuretics; reduces systemic meningeal edema and elevated serum glucose levels As emergency treatment of undiagnosed coma For administration of intravenous medications	Provides an easily metabolized source of calories (monosaccharides and disaccharides) Dextrose is oxidized to yield water in the body Higher concentrated solutions decrease glycogen content of the liver, act as protein sparer, and prevent steratic ketosis; may cause glycosuria and osmotic diuresis	CHF Circulatory insufficiency Kidney dysfunction Hypoproteinemia Head injuries Diabetes Not for subcutaneous injection

(cont'd.)

Intravenous Solution	Uses	Action and Fate	Relative Contraindications
COMBINATION SALINE AND DEXTROSE SOLUTIONS (per liter)			
–5% dextrose in 0.2 NaCl (isotonic) (38 mEq Na^+, 38 mEq Cl, 170 calories) –5% dextrose in 0.33 NaCl (hypertonic) (56 mEq Na^+, 56 mEq Cl, 170 calories) –5% dextrose in 0.45 NaCl (hypertonic) (77 mEq Na^+, 77 mEq Cl, 170 calories)	Prepared in combination for individual needs relating to the patient's condition Fluid maintenance/replacement with both calories and electrolytes	Same as those of saline and dextrose solutions combined	CHF Circulatory insufficiency Kidney dysfunction Hypoproteinemia Diabetes Head injuries Hypernatremia Not for subcutaneous injection

–5% dextrose in 0.9 NaCl (hypertonic) (154 mEq Na^+, 154 mEq Cl, 170 calories)

–5% dextrose in Lactated Ringer's (hypertonic) (130 mEq Na^+, 109 mEq Cl, 4 mEq K^+, 3 mg Ca^{++}, 28 mg HCO_3, 170 calories)

(cont'd.)

Intravenous Solution	Uses	Action and Fate	Relative Contraindications
PLASMA AND SERUM REPLACEMENT SOLUTIONS			
–Plasmolate (Plasma Protein Fraction, USP) (5% solution) –Salt-poor serum albumin (25% solution) (isotonic) See monograph albumin, normal serum	Hypovolemic shock Nephrosis and other conditions in which hypoproteinemia exists	Blood volume expander (Plasmolate): oncotic action approximately equivalent to that of human plasma Does not produce any additional oxygen-carrying ability Contains no clotting elements	CHF Severe anemia Hepatic disease or failure Low calorie reserve

Part Three
Drug Monographs

Drugs are listed alphabetically according to GENERIC NAMES, followed by common trade names.

ACEBUTOLOL Sectral

CLASS
–Beta-adrenergic blocker (antihypertensive; antidysrhythmic)

USES
–Mild-to-moderate hypertension
–Sinus tachycardia
–Treatment of ventricular dysrhythmias
–Prophylaxis of angina pectoris

ACTION
–Completely blocks stimulation of beta-adrenergic receptors within vascular smooth muscle to lower blood pressure
–Decreases rate of SA node discharge, slows conduction of AV node, and increases recovery time, which all act to decrease O_2 demand in the myocardium

USUAL DOSAGE/ROUTE

ADULT
–PO: 400–800 mg/day, single dose or twice daily (up to 1200 mg/day)

PEDIATRIC
–Not for use in children

ADVERSE/SIDE EFFECTS

RAPID
–Dizziness
–Bradycardia
–Congestive heart failure
–Rash
–Bronchospasm
–Profound hypotension
–2d- and 3d-degree heart block
–Cold extremities
–N & V

GRADUAL
–Fatigue
–Weakness
–Depression
–Mental changes
–Pulmonary edema
–Impotence
–Joint pain
–Diarrhea
–Agranulocytosis
–Thrombocytopenia

CONTRAINDICATIONS
–Hypersensitivity to beta blockers
–Uncompensated heart failure
–Pulmonary edema
–Cardiogenic shock
–Bradycardia heart block

SPECIAL PRECAUTIONS
–Pregnant or lactating patients
–Renal impairment (dosage reduction necessary)
–Elderly patients (increased sensitivity to the effects)
–Major surgery
–Diabetes mellitus
–Thyroid disease
–COPD
–Asthma

OTHER SPECIAL INFORMATION
–Obtain baselines of renal function and liver function before therapy begins.
–Monitor blood pressure during beginning treatment and periodically thereafter for hypotensive effects.
–Take apical/radial pulse before administration.
–Caution patient that drug may cause increased sensitivity to light.
–Caution patient to avoid alcohol, smoking, and sodium intake while taking this drug.

ANTIDOTE

SEVERE REACTIONS

–D/C drug immediately and initiate appropriate treatment for symptoms.

–Treat overdose with lavage, then ATROPINE IV for bradycardia; THEOPHYLLINE IV for bronchospasm; glucose IV for hypoglycemia; DIAZEPAM IV for seizures.

–Treat cardiac failure with a diuretic, DIGITALIS, oxygen, and hemodialysis.

–Treat hypotension with a vasopressor such as DOPAMINE.

OTHER REACTIONS

–Notify physician of any side effects and initiate appropriate actions.

ACETOHEXAMIDE Dimelor, Dymelor

CLASS

–Oral hypoglycemic (first-generation sulfonylurea antidiabetic)

USES

–For treatment of stable maturity-onset noninsulin-dependent diabetes mellitus (type II), uncontrolled by diet and exercise alone

ACTION

–Stimulates beta cells of pancreas to secrete insulin

–Increases receptor sites for insulin on cell walls

USUAL DOSAGE/ROUTE

ADULT

–Initially 250 mg PO daily before breakfast; may increase dose every 5–7 days (250–500 mg) as needed, not to exceed 1.5 gm daily, divided 2 times/day before the morning and evening meal

PEDIATRIC
–Not for use in children

ADVERSE/SIDE EFFECTS

RAPID
–Rashes
–Erythema, itching
–Hypoglycemia

GRADUAL
–Headache
–Weakness, fatigue
–N & V, epigastric fullness
–Heartburn
–Diarrhea
–Hepatitis
–Photosensitivity
–Aplastic anemia
–Dizziness

CONTRAINDICATIONS
–Hypersensitivity to oral hypoglycemics (sulfonylureas)
–Hyperglycemia due to primary renal disease
–Juvenile or brittle diabetes
–Pregnancy

SPECIAL PRECAUTIONS
–Elderly
–Cardiac disease
–Renal disease
–Hepatic disease
–Thyroid disease
–Severe hypoglycemic reactions
–Testosterone, cold remedies, mood elevators, sulfa drugs, salicylates, and oral anticoagulants may potentiate hypoglycemia reactions

OTHER SPECIAL INFORMATION
–Dosage must be individualized; patients who do not respond to 1.5 gm daily will generally not respond to higher doses.

–Administer 30 min before meals to diminish GI disturbances.
–Onset = 1 hr; peak = 2–3 hr; half-life = 6 hr; duration = 12–18 hr.
–Drug is metabolized in the liver.
–Over 80% of the drug is excreted in the urine.
–Test capillary blood glucose and urine glucose levels at least daily while on this drug.
–The drug must be continued on a daily basis and taken in the morning to prevent abrupt changes in the blood glucose levels.
–Avoid the use of alcohol while on this drug (decreases effectiveness and may cause an antabuse-like reaction.

ANTIDOTE

SEVERE REACTIONS
–D/C drug immediately and initiate appropriate treatment for symptoms.
–Correct overdose of drug with 10–50% glucose solution.

OTHER REACTIONS
–Notify physician of any side effects and initiate appropriate actions.

ADENOSINE Adenocard

CLASS
–Antidysrhythmic

USES
–Paroxysmal supraventricular tachycardia

ACTION
–Slows AV node conduction by interrupting reentry pathways to AV node, restores normal sinus rhythm

USUAL DOSAGE/ROUTE

ADULT

–IV bolus: 6 mg, then if unconverted within 1–2 min, 12 mg by rapid IV bolus; may repeat 12-mg dose again

PEDIATRIC

–Safe use in children not established

ADVERSE/SIDE EFFECTS

RAPID

–Nausea
–Metallic taste
–Throat tightness
–Groin pressure
–Dyspnea, chest pressure, hyperventilation
–Light-headedness
–Dizziness
–Arm tingling
–Numbness
–Chest pain
–Atrial tachydysrhythmia
–Palpitations
–Hypotension

GRADUAL

–Apprehension
–Blurred vision
–Headache
–Sweating

CONTRAINDICATIONS

–Hypersensitivity
–2nd- or 3rd-degree heart block
–AV block
–Sick sinus syndrome
–Atrial flutter
–Atrial fibrillation
–Ventricular tachycardia

SPECIAL PRECAUTIONS
–Pregnant or lactating patients
–Children
–Asthma

OTHER SPECIAL INFORMATION
–DIPYRIDAMOLE increases drug action.
–CNS stimulants (Methylxanthines) such as THEOPHYLLINE and caffeine decrease, antagonize the action of this drug.

ANTIDOTE

SEVERE REACTIONS
–D/C drug immediately and initiate appropriate treatment for symptoms.
–Defibrillate.
–Administer vasopressor such as DOPAMINE, ISOPROTERENOL for hypotension.

OTHER REACTIONS
–Notify physician of any side effects and initiate appropriate actions.

ALBUMIN, NORMAL SERUM Albuminar, Albumisol, Albutein, Buminate, Plasbumin

CLASS
–Parenteral protein, blood derivative

USES
–Shock, regardless of etiology
–Hyperbilirubinemia (binds bilirubin)
–Hypoproteinemia
–Burns for the correction of fluid losses
–Prevention and treatment of cerebral edema
–Varicella zoster infections (supportive treatment)

ACTION

–Maintains colloid osmotic pressure of the plasma
–Restores and exposes plasma volume of circulating blood by mobilizing fluid from extravascular tissue into intravascular space
–Nourishes tissue

USUAL DOSAGE/ROUTE

ADULT AND PEDIATRIC (over 12 years)

5% SOLUTION

–*Burns:* 100–200 ml
–*Shock:* Initially 250–500 ml; repeated doses every 30 min depending on response to initial dose

25% IV INFUSION SOLUTION

–*Shock:* 100–200 ml followed by 100 ml as needed dependent on blood pressure
–*Hypoproteinemia:* 200–300 ml
–*Cerebral edema:* 60–80 ml infused in 8–10 min

PEDIATRIC (under 12 years)

–*Shock:* 125–250 ml of 5% sol every 30 min as needed until desirable blood pressure is obtained
–*Burns:* 2.2 ml/kg of 5% sol in normal saline (NS) (mix 40 ml albumin in 160 ml NS for administration)
–*Hypoproteinemia:* 6–25 gm of 25% sol daily not to exceed 1 ml/min, titrated to patient response; D/C when desired effect is obtained
–*Hyperbilirubinemia* (infant): 1 gm/kg IV of 25% sol before transfusion

ADVERSE/SIDE EFFECTS

RAPID

–Chills, fever
–Hypotension
–Congestive heart failure (CHF) and pulmonary edema (PE)
–Tachycardia
–N & V

GRADUAL

–Headache
–Urticaria, rash
–Increased salivation
–Back pain
–Fever, chills, flushing

CONTRAINDICATIONS

–Hypersensitivity
–Severe anemia
–Normal or increased intravascular volume
–CHF or PE
–Allergic reactions to albumin

SPECIAL PRECAUTIONS

–Severe hepatic disease
–Severe renal disease
–Dehydrated (additional fluids may be required)
–Hemorrhaging and deficiency of oxygen-carrying capacity from RBC loss

OTHER SPECIAL INFORMATION

–Do not add any medication to a solution of albumin.
–25% albumin draws 3.5 times its own volume into the blood from tissues within 15 minutes of infusion.
–IV onset = 15–30 min; peak and duration is unknown.
–Infuse undiluted solution 1–2 ml/min in patients with normal blood volume to prevent fluid overload.
–Complete infusions within 4 hr.
–Compatible with D_5W, $D_{10}W$, NS, and hyperalimentation solution.
–Infusion rate for children is usually ¼–½ the adult rate of approx. 1–4 ml/min.
–Monitor for cyanosis or pallor, which may indicate reductions in the oxygen-carrying capacity of blood secondary to hemodilution.
–Monitor I & O ratio; urinary output may decrease.
–100 ml of normal serum albumin 25% provides the plasma protein of approx. 500 ml of plasma, or 2 pints of whole blood.

ANTIDOTE

SEVERE REACTIONS

–D/C drug immediately and initiate appropriate treatment for symptoms.
–Correct hemodilution by giving whole blood or packed red blood cells.
–Correct hypotension with fluid replacement.

OTHER REACTIONS

–Notify physician of any side effects and initiate appropriate actions.
–Use a new lot of drug if patient reacts to the drug but requires reinstitution.

ALBUTEROL Proventil, Ventolin

CLASS

–Adrenergic beta-2 agonist

USES

–Prevention of exercise-induced asthma
–Bronchospasm associated with bronchitis or emphysema

ACTION

–Bronchodilation by stimulation of beta-2 receptors
–Vascular and uterine smooth muscle dilatation

USUAL DOSAGE/ROUTE

ADULT

–*Asthma:* Inhalant, 2 puffs 15 min before exercising
–*Bronchospasm:* Inhalant, 1–2 puffs every 4–6 hr
–PO: 2–4 mg 3–4 times/day not to exceed 8 mg in 24 hr

PEDIATRIC

–5 mg by nebulization or IPPB 3–4 times daily

ADVERSE/SIDE EFFECTS

RAPID

–Dizziness
–Headache
–Tremors
–Anxiety
–Palpitations
–Tachycardia
–Bronchospasm

GRADUAL

–Hallucinations
–Flushing
–Irritability
–Dry nose, irritation of nose, throat
–Hypertension, angina, dysrhythmias
–Muscle cramps
–Difficulty with urination
–Heartburn
–N & V

CONTRAINDICATIONS

–Hypersensitivity to sympathomimetics
–Tachydysrhythmias
–Severe cardiac disease

SPECIAL PRECAUTIONS

–Pregnant or lactating patients
–Cardiac disorders
–Hyperthyroidism
–Diabetes mellitus
–Hypertension
–Prostatic hypertrophy
–Narrow-angle glaucoma
–Seizures

OTHER SPECIAL INFORMATION

–Tricyclic antidepressants, MAO inhibitors may increase action.
–Other beta blockers may inhibit action.

–Shake inhaler before using.
–Wait one minute between inhalations.
–Sip water between inhalant doses to help reduce dry mouth.
–Do not use other over-the-counter inhalants with this drug.

ANTIDOTE

SEVERE REACTIONS

–D/C drug immediately and initiate appropriate treatment for symptoms.
–Treat overdose with a beta-2 adrenergic blocker such as PROPRANOLOL.

OTHER REACTIONS

–Notify physician of any side effects, such as chest pain, dizziness, diaphoresis, palpitations, and initiate appropriate actions.

ALPRAZOLAM Xanax

CLASS

–Antianxiety

USES

–Short-term relief of anxiety, panic disorders

ACTION

–CNS depression of short duration

USUAL DOSAGE/ROUTE

ADULT

–PO: 0.25–0.5 mg 3 times/day, with a maximum dose of 4 mg/day in divided doses

PEDIATRIC

–Not recommended for children under 18 years

ADVERSE/SIDE EFFECTS

RAPID

–Dizziness
–Drowsiness
–Orthostatic hypotension
–Blurred vision
–Rash
–Dermatitis
–Dry mouth

GRADUAL

–Constipation
–Anorexia

CONTRAINDICATIONS

–Hypersensitivity
–Narrow-angle glaucoma
–Pregnancy

SPECIAL PRECAUTIONS

–Hepatic disease
–Renal disease
–Debilitation
–Elderly may need decreased dosage
–Alcohol consumption

OTHER SPECIAL INFORMATION

–Administer with food or milk.
–Monitor BP, liver function, renal function.
–Hard candy or gum may help reduce dry mouth.

ANTIDOTE

SEVERE REACTIONS

–D/C drug immediately and initiate appropriate treatment for symptoms.
–Treat overdose with gastric lavage.

OTHER REACTIONS

–Notify physician of any side effects and initiate appropriate actions.

AMINOCAPROIC ACID Amicar

CLASS

–Fibrinolysis inhibitor (hemostatic that checks blood flow)

USES

–Excessive bleeding from systemic hyperfibrinolysis and urinary fibrinolysis
–Abruptio placenta
–Adjunctive therapy in hemophilia
–Surgical bleeding following surgery (heart, lung, prostate, cervix, stomach, and other) with heavy bleeding
–Antidote for thrombolytic agents

ACTION

–Inhibits plasminogen activator substances, thus inhibiting fibrinolysis and stabilizing of clot formation.

USUAL DOSAGE/ROUTE

ADULT

–PO or IV: Initial dose 4–5 gm over first hour, followed by 1.0–1.25-gm doses at hourly intervals, not exceeding 30 gm in any 24–hour period

PEDIATRIC

–100 mg/kg or 3 gm/M^2 over first hr, followed by continuous infusion of 33.3 mg/kg/hr or 1 gm/M^2/hr, not exceeding 18 gm/M^2/24 hr.

ADVERSE/SIDE EFFECTS

RAPID

–NVD
–Dysrhythmias
–Postural hypotension
–Diuresis, renal failure

GRADUAL

–Nasal stuffiness
–Skin rash

–Anorexia
–Malaise
–Headache

CONTRAINDICATIONS
–Hypersensitivity
–Should not be used with evidence of an active intravascular clotting process
–Postpartum bleeding
–DIC (disseminated intravascular coagulation)
–New burns
–Patients on estrogens or oral contraceptives

SPECIAL PRECAUTIONS
–Hematuria originating in the upper urinary tract
–Cardiac disease (dosage reduction required)
–Liver disease (dosage reduction required)
–Renal disease (dosage reduction required)
–Thrombosis
–Pregnancy and lactation

OTHER SPECIAL INFORMATION
–For IV infusion, dilute with 250 ml sterile water, NS, D_5W or Ringer's solution.
–Rapid IV infusion may cause hypotension, bradycardia, or dysrhythmias.
–Monitor VS frequently while administering the drug.
–Assess for thromboembolic complications.
–PO and IV drug peaks in 2 hr and is excreted by the kidneys.

ANTIDOTE

SEVERE REACTIONS
–D/C drug immediately and initiate appropriate treatment for symptoms.

OTHER REACTIONS
–Notify physician of any side effects and initiate appropriate actions.

AMINOPHYLLINE, THEOPHYLLINE, ETHYLENEDIAMINE Lixaminol, Phyllocontin, Somophyllin

CLASS
–Bronchodilator, smooth muscle relaxant

USES
–Bronchospasm
–Bronchial asthma
–Bronchitis

ACTION
–Relaxes respiratory system smooth muscle

USUAL DOSAGE/ROUTE

ADULT
–PO: 500 mg, then 250–500 mg every 6–8 hr
–IV infusion: 0.3–0.9 mg/kg/hr (peak = 30 min)
–Rectally: 500 mg every 6–8 hr

PEDIATRIC
–PO: 7.5 mg/kg, then 3–6 mg/kg every 6–8 hr
–IV: 7.5 mg/kg, then 3–6 mg/kg every 6–8 hr infused over 5 min. Do not exceed 25 mg/min.
–IV infusion: 1 mg/kg/hr

ADVERSE/SIDE EFFECTS

RAPID
–Anxiety
–Restlessness
–N & V
–Dizziness
–Convulsion
–Sinus tachycardia
–Hypotension

GRADUAL
–Diarrhea
–Headache
–Insomnia

CONTRAINDICATIONS
–Hypersensitivity
–Tachydysrhythmias

SPECIAL PRECAUTIONS
–Elderly
–Children
–Liver disease
–Peptic ulcer disease
–Diabetes mellitus
–Hypertension
–Hyperthyroidism

OTHER SPECIAL INFORMATION
–Do not mix with other medication in a syringe.
–Drug may alter effect of anticoagulants.
–Drug action may increase if administered with CIMETIDINE, PROPRANOLOL.
–Monitor ERYTHROMYCIN blood levels of drug.
–Administer po after meals.

ANTIDOTE

SEVERE REACTIONS
–D/C drug immediately and initiate appropriate treatment for symptoms.

OTHER REACTIONS
–Notify physician of any side effects and initiate appropriate actions.

AMMONIA, AROMATIC SPIRIT Aromatic Ammonia Spirit

CLASS
–Respiratory stimulant

USES
–Treatment and prevention of syncopal episodes

ACTION
–Irritation to nasal, esophageal, and gastric mucosa
–Stimulates respiratory and vasomotor centers of the medulla

USUAL DOSAGE/ROUTE
ADULT
–Inhalation of 1 capsule after breakage for syncopy
–PO: 2–4 ml diluted in 30–45 ml of water

PEDIATRIC
–Not recommended for pediatric use

ADVERSE/SIDE EFFECTS
RAPID
–Increase in BP

GRADUAL
–None known

CONTRAINDICATIONS
–None known

SPECIAL PRECAUTIONS
–COPD or asthma

SPECIAL INFORMATION
–Be sure patient has inhaled enough of the vapor to elicit a response.
–Stand clear of patient when using spirit; patient may respond

suddenly and violently in attempt to escape the occurring respiratory irritation.
–Do not place inhalation packets in pockets. They may open and cause caustic burns.
–Evaluate the original cause of the syncopal episode.

ANTIDOTE

SEVERE REACTIONS

–D/C drug immediately and intiate treatment for symptoms.

OTHER REACTIONS

–Notify physician of any side effects and initiate appropriate actions.

AMOXICILLIN TRIHYDRATE Amoxil, Larotid, Polymox, Trimox, Wymox, and others

CLASS

–Broad-spectrum antibiotics

USES

–Pneumonia
–Sinus infections
–Urinary tract infections
–Mastoiditis
–Meningitis

ACTION

–Interferes with bacterial cell wall synthesis

USUAL DOSAGE/ROUTE

ADULT

–PO: 250–500 mg every 8 hr

PEDIATRIC

–PO: 20–40 mg/kg/day in divided doses every 8 hr

ADVERSE/SIDE EFFECTS

RAPID

–Anaphylaxis
–Rash
–NVD

GRADUAL

–Glomerulonephritis
–Colitis
–Oliguria
–Hematuria
–Bone marrow suppression

CONTRAINDICATIONS

–Sensitivity to PENICILLINS
–Use in neonates

SPECIAL PRECAUTIONS

–Pregnant or lactating patients
–Hypersensitivity to CEPHALOSPORINS

OTHER SPECIAL INFORMATION

–Monitor liver and renal studies.
–Take drug in equal intervals around the clock to maintain blood levels.

ANTIDOTE

SEVERE REACTIONS

–D/C drug immediately and initiate appropriate treatment for symptoms.
–Treat anaphylaxis with EPINEPHRINE, AMINOPHYLLINE, O_2, IV corticosteroids, antihistamines, and ALS procedures as needed.

OTHER REACTIONS

–Notify physician of any side effects and initiate appropriate actions.

AMYL NITRATE, USP Amyl Nitrate Inhalation

CLASS
–Coronary vasodilator

USES
–Angina pectoris
–Cyanide poisoning antidote

ACTION
–Relaxes all smooth muscles (vascular, GI, etc.), resulting in reduced vascular resistance
–Coronary artery dilator
–Reduces cardiac output, preload and afterload

USUAL DOSAGE/ROUTE
ADULT
–*Angina pectoris:* Inhalation 0.18–0.3 ml (one ampule) as needed; may repeat in 3–5 min.
–*Cyanide poisoning:* Inhalation 0.3 ml ampule every 15–30 sec until IV sodium nitrite infusion is available (see AHFS 24:12)

PEDIATRIC
–Safe use in children not established

ADVERSE/SIDE EFFECTS
RAPID
–Headache
–Postural hypotension
–Tachycardia
–Flushing of face, pallor
–Dizziness
–Cold sweat
–N & V
–Syncope
–Weakness
–Respiratory depression and apnea

GRADUAL

–None known

CONTRAINDICATIONS

–Hypersensitivity to nitrites
–Severe anemia
–Hypertension
–Glaucoma
–Increased intracranial pressure
–Acute myocardial infarction

SPECIAL PRECAUTIONS

–Pregnant and lactating patients
–Drug abuse patients
–Recent head injury/trauma
–Cerebral hemorrhage
–Hypotension
–Hypovolemic patients
–Cardiac tamponade or constrictive pericarditis

OTHER SPECIAL INFORMATION

–This drug is more likely to produce headache and lowered blood pressure than other nitrite preparations.
–Vapors are highly flammable.
–Have patient sit while administering because of the high incidence of postural hypotension.
–Street drug of abuse; street term is "neohigh."
–Onset = 30 sec; half-life = 1–4 min; duration = 3–5 min.

ANTIDOTE

SEVERE REACTIONS

–D/C drug immediately and initiate appropriate treatment for symptoms.
–Treat hypotension with vasopressor such as DOPAMINE.

OTHER REACTIONS

–Notify physician of any side effects and initiate appropriate actions.

ANISTREPLASE (APSAC) Eminase

CLASS
–Thrombolytic enzyme

USES
–Management of acute myocardial infarction

ACTION
–Promotes thrombolysis, promotes conversion of plasminogen to plasmin

USUAL DOSAGE/ROUTE
ADULT
–IV: 30 units over 4–5 min as soon as possible after onset of symptoms (30 units per vial); reconstitute vial with 5 ml sterile water

PEDIATRIC
–Safe use in children not established

ADVERSE/SIDE EFFECTS
RAPID
–Bronchospasm
–Anaphylaxis
–Bleeding
–Dyspnea
–Hypotension
–Reperfusion dysrhythmias

GRADUAL
–Headache
–Tremor
–Intracranial bleeding
–Retroperitoneal bleeding
–Surface bleeding
–N & V

CONTRAINDICATIONS
–Hypersensitivity
–Active bleeding
–CNS neoplasms
–Cerebral hemorrhage
–Cerebral embolism/thrombosis
–Severe hypertension
–Recent surgery, especially intraspinal or intracranial
–Recent intraarterial diagnostic procedure

SPECIAL PRECAUTIONS
–Pregnant patients
–Hepatic disease
–Renal disease
–Ulcerative colitis
–COPD
–Cardiovascular disorders such as rheumatic valve disease, left heart arterial emboli, or subacute bacterial endocarditis

OTHER SPECIAL INFORMATION
–Half-life = 105–120 min.
–Drug is most effective if given within 30 min of onset of symptoms.
–Monitor vital signs closely.
–Monitor Hct, platelets, PTT, PT, APTT frequently after use.
–Avoid other invasive procedures during therapy.
–Follow drug with HEPARIN therapy in 4–6 hr.
–Reconstitute with sterile water only and roll (not shake) to reconstitute.

ANTIDOTE

SEVERE REACTIONS
–D/C drug immediately and initiate appropriate treatment for symptoms.
–Use cryoprecipitate or fresh frozen plasma for bleeding.

OTHER REACTIONS
–Notify physician of any side effects and initiate appropriate actions.
–Treat rash with antihistamines.

ATENOLOL Tenormin

CLASS
–Antihypertensive, synthetic beta-adrenergic receptor blocking agent, antianginal

USES
–Management of hypertension, alone or with other antihypertensive agents, particularly thiazide-type diuretics
–Management of angina pectoris

ACTION
–Blocks stimulation of beta-1 (myocardial) adrenergic receptors to decrease blood pressure and heart rate, and thereby lowering myocardial oxygen consumption

USUAL DOSAGE/ROUTE
ADULT
–Initially 50 mg/day PO, progressing to 50–150 mg/day
PEDIATRIC
–Safe use in children not established

ADVERSE/SIDE EFFECTS
RAPID
–Profound hypotension
–Bradycardia
–2nd- and 3rd-degree heart block
–Postural hypotension
–Bronchospasm, wheezing, dyspnea
–Dizziness
–Drowsiness
GRADUAL
–CHF
–Cold extremities
–Insomnia
–Fatigue, tiredness
–Depression

–Strange dreams
–Catatonia
–Diarrhea
–N & V
–Agranulocytosis
–Alopecia
–Dry throat and eyes
–Impotence

CONTRAINDICATIONS

–Hypersensitivity to beta-blockers
–Sinus bradycardia
–Greater than first-degree heart block
–Overt cardiac failure
–Cardiogenic shock
–Bronchospastic disease
–CHF

SPECIAL PRECAUTIONS

–Pregnant and lactating patients
–Following surgery
–Diabetes mellitus
–Renal disease
–Thyroid disease
–COPD, asthma

OTHER SPECIAL INFORMATION

–Caution patient about side effects.
–Advise patient to have blood pressure checked regularly for decreases.
–Onset = 1 hr; peak = 2–4 hr; duration = 24 hr.
–Drug may mask clinical signs of hyperthyroidism or hypoglycemia.
–Hold drug if apical pulse is less than 50 bpm and notify physician.

ANTIDOTE

SEVERE REACTIONS

–D/C drug immediately and initiate appropriate treatment for symptoms.

–Lavage patient's stomach to remove residual drug.
–Treat bradycardia with ATROPINE.
–Treat bronchospasm with THEOPHYLLINE, DIGITALIS, OXYGEN.
–Treat cardiac failure with DIURETICS.
–Consider the need for hemodialysis.

OTHER REACTIONS
–Notify physician of any side effects and initiate appropriate actions.

ATROPINE SULFATE Atropine

CLASS
–Anticholinergic

USES
–Bradydysrhythmias
–Bradycardia
–Asystole
–Decreases secretions before and during surgery
–Spastic conditions of GI tract and peptic ulcers
–Antispasmotic with GU conditions
–Nerve gas poisoning and mushroom poisoning
–Anticholinesterase, insecticide poisoning
–Dilation of pupil (mydriatics)
–Antidote for physostigmine and pilocarpine

ACTION
–Blocks acetylcholine and antagonizes histamine and serotonin, thereby blocking vagal stimulation and increasing the rate of discharge of the SA node (increased heart rate)
–Inhibits smooth muscles and glands affected by postganglionic cholinergic nerves
–Blocks vagus nerve and dries secretions

USUAL DOSAGE/ROUTE

ADULT (route, SC, IM, IV)

–IV: 0.5 mg every 5 min up to 2 mg for sinus bradycardia with decreased BP and complete heart block
–IM: 0.4–0.6 mg or SC 30–60 min preoperatively

PEDIATRIC (route, SC, IM, IV)

–IV: 0.01–0.02 mg/kg/IV up to 0.4 mg; or 0.3 mg/M^2 and may repeat dose as needed every 4–6 hr
–IM/SC: 0.1–0.4 mg IM or SC 30–60 min preoperatively
–Minimum dose is 0.1 mg to prevent paradoxical bradycardia

ADVERSE/SIDE EFFECTS

RAPID

–Flushing, dry and warm skin
–N & V
–Dryness of nasopharyngeal and oral mucous membranes
–Confusion, anxiety
–Dilated pupils
–Angina
–PVCs
–Headache, drowsiness
–Hypotension

GRADUAL

–Impotence
–Dysuria
–Retention
–Hesitancy
–Anorexia
–Constipation
–Paralytic ileus

CONTRAINDICATIONS

–Hypersensitivity
–Glaucoma
–Prostatic hypertrophy
–Ulcerative colitis
–Paralytic ileus, pyloric stenosis, GI obstructions
–Tachycardia/tachydysrhythmias
–Asthma

SPECIAL PRECAUTIONS

–Pregnant and lactating patients
–Renal disease
–Hyperthyroidism
–Liver disease
–Patients under age 6
–COPD

OTHER SPECIAL INFORMATION

–Postural hypotension can occur from use of the drug.
–Urinary retention may occur.
–Risk of heat stroke is increased by suppressing perspiration.
–Atropine is usually the only preanesthetic required in infants less than 6 months of age.
–Hypersensitivity is possible in children with Down's syndrome.

ANTIDOTE

SEVERE REACTIONS

–D/C drug immediately and initiate appropriate treatment for symptoms.
–Treat hypotension with vasopressors such as DOPAMINE.
–Treat convulsions with DIAZEPAM.
–Treat dysrhythmias with antidysrhythmias such as LIDOCAINE.

OTHER REACTIONS

–Notify physician of any side effects and initiate appropriate actions.
–Administer oxygen.
–Monitor EKG.

BENZTROPINE MESYLATE Apo-Benzotropine, Bensylate, Cogentin, PMS Benzotropine

CLASS
–Anticholinergic (antiparkinsonian agent)

USES
–Parkinsonism
–Extrapyramidal muscle movement and rigidity reactions to antipsychotic drugs
–Oculogyric crisis due to postencephalitic parkinsonism or encephalitis lethargia

ACTION
–Reduces extrapyramidal muscle movements by blocking excess CNS cholinergic receptors that are associated with dopamine deficiency in the basal ganglia, and by blocking dopamine reuptake and storage at central receptor sites

USUAL DOSAGE/ROUTE

ADULT
–*Parkinsonism:* PO: 0.5–1.0 mg initially, increasing gradually as tolerated up to a max. of 6 mg/day
–*Extrapyramidal reactions:* PO, IM, IV: 1–2 mg IM or IV initially, followed by 1–2 mg PO twice/day to prevent recurrence

PEDIATRIC
–Safe use in children under age 3 not established, otherwise use lower dosing protocols as for adults

ADVERSE/SIDE EFFECTS

RAPID
–Tachycardia
–Palpitations
–Rash
–Dry mouth

–N & V
–Dizziness
–Muscle weakness
–Blurred vision
–Parasthesia
–Dilated pupils

GRADUAL
–Constipation
–Epigastric distress
–Restlessness
–Irritability
–Hallucinations
–Confusion
–Memory loss
–Photophobia
–Urinary retention
–Decreased sweating
–Headache
–Depression

CONTRAINDICATIONS
–Hypersensitivity
–Pregnant or lactating patients
–Narrow-angle glaucoma
–GI obstructive disease
–Urinary tract obstruction
–Tardive dyskinesia
–Children under 3 yr

SPECIAL PRECAUTIONS
–Tachycardia
–Prostatic hypertrophy
–Elderly
–Young children

OTHER SPECIAL INFORMATION
–Reduction in the dosage is required for this drug when used in conjunction with AMANTADINE, alcohol, antihistamine, narcotics, sedatives, hypnotics, phenothiazines, and

antidepressants (these drugs increase CNS depression and anticholinergic effects).
- –This drug enhances the effect of LEVODOPA and SINEMET.
- –Give with food or after meals to reduce GI symptoms.
- –Do not abruptly discontinue this drug.
- –Discontinue drug if the following hypersensitive signs/symptoms occur: urinary retention, confusion, hallucinations, dilated and nonreactive pupils, hot and dry flushed skin.
- –Oculogyric crisis is an involuntary attack of deviation and fixation of the eyeballs, usually upward, that may last several minutes to several hours.

ANTIDOTE

SEVERE REACTIONS
- –D/C drug immediately and initiate appropriate treatment for symptoms.
- –Treat overdose with the antidote PHYSOSTIGMINE.
- –Treat shock with IV fluids.
- –Treat psychotic symptoms with DIAZEPAM.

OTHER REACTIONS
- –Notify physician of any side effects and initiate appropriate actions.
- –Treat urinary retention with foley catheterization.
- –Treat mydriasis of the eyes with PILOCARPINE drops.
- –Treat other reactions symptomatically.

BLOOD (WHOLE/PACKED RED BLOOD CELLS) Whole Blood; PRBCs

CLASS
- –Whole blood and blood components (whole blood contains RBCs, plasma, plasma proteins, and 63 ml per 500 ml bag of an anticoagulant/preservative solution; PRBCs contain RBCs [80%], plasma [20%], in a total volume of 250–350 ml per unit)

USES

–Whole blood: Acute or massive blood loss (hypovolemic shock) greater than or equal to 1/3 of the client's total blood volume (adult = 1000–1200 ml)

–PRBCs: Restoration or maintenance of adequate organ oxygenation with minimal expansion of intravascular blood volume in anemia

ACTION

–Red blood cells increase oxygen-carrying properties, and plasma provides for intravascular volume expansion.

USUAL DOSAGE/ROUTE

ADULT

–*Whole blood:* The average dose is determined by the clinical situation.

–*PRBCs:* Average dose is 2 units, but is determined by the clinical situation.

PEDIATRIC

–*Whole blood and PRBCs:* The average dose is determined by the clinical situation.

ADVERSE/SIDE EFFECTS

RAPID

–Anaphylaxis
–High fever
–Hemolytic reaction
–Chills
–Dyspnea
–Cough
–Urticaria
–Flushing
–Asthmatic wheeze
–Laryngeal edema
–Anxiety
–Headache
–Low back pain
–Tachycardia

–Tachypnea
–Hypotension (vascular collapse)

GRADUAL
–Circulatory overload
–Crackles at base of lungs
–NVD
–Hypertension
–Hypotension (septic reaction)
–Distended neck veins
–Bleeding
–Acute renal failure
–Blood in urine
–Delayed hemolytic reaction

CONTRAINDICATIONS
–Hypersensitivity
–CHF and PE
–Systemic infection process with elevated temperature
–Jehovah's Witness (religion) unless consent verified

SPECIAL PRECAUTIONS
–COPD clients
–Hypertensive disease
–Previous allergic reactions to infusion
–Children and infants
–Elderly

OTHER SPECIAL INFORMATION
–Use a 19G or larger bore needle and a small-pore filter when infusing.
–Flush IV tubing before and after infusion with 0.9 NaCL.
–PRBCs may be viscous and require dilution with 0.9 NaCL.
–Confirm ABO blood type and Rh compatibility, as well as client identification prior to administration.
–Infuse each unit IV over 2–3 hr but complete the unit in a 4-hr period (too fast an infusion may hemolyze RBCs, and may increase the risk for reactions and/or fluid overload).
–Warm the blood (less than or equal to 39°C) whenever possible to prevent hypothermia and cardiac dysrhythmias.

–Observe clients for fluid overload (increased venous pressure, distended neck veins, dyspnea, cough, crackles at base of lungs).
–Wear protective gloves and clothing to prevent spread of hepatitis and/or viruses.
–Observe clients for diseases that may be transmitted by blood transfusion (hepatitis, malaria, syphilis, AIDS, graft-versus-host disease).
–Clean any blood spill with a 1:10 solution of bleach or other antimicrobial.
–Donor compatibility is as follows:

Whole blood:	A recipient from A donor
	B recipient from B donor
	O recipient from O donor
	AB recipient from AB donor
	Rh positive recipient from Rh positive or negative donor
	Rh negative recipient from Rh negative donor
PRBCs:	A recipient from A or O donor
	B recipient from B or O donor
	O recipient from O donor
	AB recipient from A or B or O or AB donor
	Rh positive recipient from Rh positive or negative donor
	RH negative recipient from Rh negative donor

ANTIDOTE

SEVERE REACTIONS

–D/C drug immediately and initiate appropriate treatment for symptoms.
–Initiate ALS protocols and resuscitate as necessary.

OTHER REACTIONS

–Notify physician of any side effects and initiate appropriate actions.
–Return blood bags and tubing to blood bank for evaluation.
–Obtain a clotted blood sample and an anticoagulated blood

sample for examination of blood type and Coombs test for antibodies.

BRETYLIUM TOSYLATE Bretylol

CLASS
—Antidysrhythmic, adrenergic blocking agent

USES
—Short-term treatment for severe ventricular dysrhythmias that are unresponsive to conventional antidysrhythmic therapy (tachycardia, cardioversion, ventricular fibrillation)

ACTION
–Believed to suppress ventricular fibrillation probably by direct effect on the myocardium by raising ventricular fibrillation threshold
–Produces an adrenergic blocking effect

USUAL DOSAGE/ROUTE
ADULT
–IV loading dose: 5 mg/kg IV undiluted with additional doses of 10 mg/kg and may repeat every 5–30 min to maximum of 30 mg/kg
–IV or IM maintenance dose: 5–10 mg/kg every 6–8 hr or 1–2 mg/min continuous diluted infusion

PEDIATRIC
–Safe use in children not established

ADVERSE/SIDE EFFECTS
RAPID
–Bradycardia
–Initial increase in dysrhythmias (PVCs)
–Hypotension
–Increased sensitivity to catecholamines

–Angina
–Respiratory depression

GRADUAL
–NVD
–Dizziness, vertigo, syncope
–Anorexia

CONTRAINDICATIONS
–Hypersensitivity
–Digitalis toxicity
–Aortic stenosis
–Pulmonary hypertension
–There are no contraindications in treatment of ventricular fibrillation in life-threatening refractory ventricular dysrhythmias.

SPECIAL PRECAUTIONS
–Pregnant and lactating patients
–Impaired renal function
–Sinus bradycardia
–Patients on digitalis maintenance

OTHER SPECIAL INFORMATION
–Drug should be diluted to 1 part drug with 4 parts dextrose injection USP, or sodium chloride injection USP before intravenous use.
–Use various sites for IM injections.

ANTIDOTE

SEVERE REACTIONS
–D/C drug immediately and initiate appropriate treatment for symptoms.
–Correct hypotension by using DOPAMINE HCL.
–Use artificial ventilation for respiratory depression.
–Treat convulsions with DIAZEPAM.

OTHER REACTIONS
–Notify physician of any side effects and initiate appropriate actions.
–Decrease N & V by reducing rate of IV administration.

BUMETANIDE Bumex

CLASS
–Loop diuretic, antihypertensive

USES
–Edema associated with congestive heart failure
–Renal disease
–Pulmonary edema
–Ascites
–Hypertension

ACTION
–In the loop of Henle, inhibits reabsorption of sodium and chloride
–Increases excretion of water, sodium, chloride, calcium, magnesium, and hydrogen from kidneys
–Lowers blood pressure

USUAL DOSAGE/ROUTE
ADULT
–PO: 0.5–2.0 mg/day, not to exceed 10 mg/day (given on alternate days or intermittently)
–IM, IV: 0.5–1.0 mg/day, may give 2nd or 3rd dose at 2–3-hr intervals, not to exceed 10 mg/day

PEDIATRIC (use with extreme caution)
–IM, IV: 0.015–0.1 mg/kg/day given every other day

ADVERSE/SIDE EFFECTS
RAPID
–Circulatory collapse
–Renal failure
–Nausea
–Hypotension

GRADUAL
–Nausea
–Muscle cramps

–Dizziness
–Rash
–Acute pancreatitis
–Jaundice
–Loss of hearing
–Stevens–Johnson syndrome
–Thrombocytopenia
–Agranulocytosis
–Neutropenia
–Hyperglycemia
–Reduced levels of potassium, chloride, magnesium, uric acid, calcium, sodium

CONTRAINDICATIONS
–Hypersensitivity to sulfonamide
–Anuria or oliguria associated with increasing BUN and creatinine levels
–Hepatic coma
–Hypovolemia
–Lactating patients
–Electrolyte depletion

SPECIAL PRECAUTIONS
–Dehydration
–Pregnancy
–Ascites
–Severe renal disease
–Children under age 18

OTHER SPECIAL INFORMATION
–Decreased diuretic effect occurs with INDOMETHACIN.
–Drug can cause ototoxicity when used with aminoglycosides or CISPLATIN.
–Effect increases when used with antihypertensives.
–Effect of antidiabetics decreases when given with this drug.
–Toxicity increases with LITHIUM and nonpolarizing skeletal muscle relaxants.
–Dilute IV push dosage with dextrose or saline and push slowly over 1–2 min.
–Give in A.M. to avoid diuresis during sleep

–Supplement potassium as needed when using this drug.
–Give with food to decrease nausea.

ANTIDOTE

SEVERE REACTIONS

–D/C drug immediately and initiate appropriate treatment for symptoms.
–For PO overdosage, lavage the stomach.
–For deviations in blood sugar or lowererd BP, administer a combination dextrose and saline solution.

OTHER REACTIONS

–Notify physician of any side effects and initiate appropriate actions.
–Replace electrolytes as needed.

BUTORPHANOL TARTRATE Stadol

CLASS

–Narcotic analgesic

USES

–Management of moderate-to-severe pain

ACTION

–Binds with opiate receptors to block pain transmission to spinal cord
–Causes CNS depression

USUAL DOSAGE/ROUTE

ADULT

–IM: 1–4 mg every 3–4 hr as needed; deep IM, rotate sites
–IV: 0.5–2.0 mg every 3–4 hr as needed given over 3–5 min

PEDIATRIC

–Use with caution in children under age 18.
–Safety in children below age 18 has not been established.

ADVERSE/SIDE EFFECTS

RAPID

–Sedation
–Confusion
–Hallucination
–Sweating
–Respiratory depression
–Hypotension

GRADUAL

–N & V
–Urinary retention
–Palpitations
–Blurred vision

CONTRAINDICATIONS

–Hypersensitivity
–Persons with narcotic dependency
–CHF
–Myocardial infarction

SPECIAL PRECAUTIONS

–Pregnant or lactating patients
–Increased intracranial pressure
–Renal disease
–Hepatic disease
–Pulmonary disease
–Elderly or debilitated patients
–Patients on MAO inhibitors

OTHER SPECIAL INFORMATION

–Patient may have addictive CNS depression if drug used with alcohol, antihistamines, and sedative/hypnotics.
–Smoking reduces effectiveness of drug.
–Drug may cause dependency, withdrawal symptoms if rapidly discontinued.
–Prevent atelectasis by frequent position changes and cough/deep breathing.

ANTIDOTE

SEVERE REACTIONS

–D/C drug immediately and initiate appropriate treatment for symptoms.

–Administer NALOXONE 0.2–0.5 mg IV.

OTHER REACTIONS

–Notify physician of any side effects and initiate appropriate actions.

CALCIUM CHLORIDE, USP, CALCIUM GLUCEPTATE, USP, CALCIUM GLUCONATE, USP Calcium Chloride, Calcium Gluconate

CLASS

–Calcium replenisher, cation electrolyte

USES

–Tetany, hypoparathyroidism, vitamin D deficiency, alkalosis, intestinal malabsorption states, cardiac toxicity of potassium
–Prevents hypocalcemia during exchange transfusions
–Antidote for magnesium sulfate intoxication
–Neonatal tetany
–Lead colic

ACTION

–Calcium is an essential element for maintenance of functional integrity of nervous, muscular, and skeletal systems, cell membrane and capillary permeability. It is an important activator in many enzyme reactions. Calcium has a positive inotropic effect on heart muscle.

USUAL DOSAGE/ROUTE

ADULT

–CHLORIDE: IV: 500 mg–1 gm every 1–3 days as indicated. Give slower than 1 ml/min.
–GLUCEPTATE: IV: 5–20 ml; IM: 2–5 ml
–GLUCONATE: PO: 1–5 gm 3 times/day; IV: 0.5–2.0 gm at 0.5 ml/min of 10% solution

PEDIATRIC

–CHLORIDE: IV: 25 mg/kg over several minutes
–GLUCEPTATE: IV: 0.5 ml/100 ml of blood for transfusion
–GLUCONATE: PO, IV: 500 mg/kg/day in divided doses

ADVERSE/SIDE EFFECTS

RAPID

–Hypercalcemia
–Cardiac arrest
–Bradycardia
–Shortened Q–T heart block
–Phlebitis with IV use

GRADUAL

–Drowsiness
–Muscle weakness
–Headache
–Constipation
–Anorexia
–N & V
–Polyuria
–Thirst

CONTRAINDICATIONS

–Hypersensitivity
–Ventricular fibrillation
–Digitalis toxicity
–Hypercalcemia
–Renal calculi

SPECIAL PRECAUTIONS

–Pregnant and lactating patients
–Renal disease
–Respiratory disease or respiratory failure
–Cor pulmonale

OTHER SPECIAL INFORMATION

–Monitor ECG when giving calcium IV.
–Severe necrosis and tissue sloughing follows extravasation of IV.
–Administer PO drug with or following meals to enhance absorption.
–Place patient on seizure precautions.

ANTIDOTE

SEVERE REACTIONS

–D/C drug immediately and initiate appropriate treatment for symptoms.

OTHER REACTIONS

–Notify physician of any side effects and initiate appropriate actions.

CAPTOPRIL Capoten

CLASS

–Angiotensin-converting enzyme (ACE) inhibitor (antihypertensive)

USES

–Hypertension

–Congestive heart failure unresponsive to conventional therapy

ACTION

–Inhibits angiotensin-converting enzyme conversion of angiotensin I to angiotensin II, decreasing arterial and venous vasoconstriction, reducing sodium retention, and lowering systemic vascular resistance, and increasing cardiac output

USUAL DOSAGE/ROUTE

ADULT

–*Hypertension:* PO: 12.5–25 mg 2–3 times/day, increasing in 25-mg increments up to a maximum of 150 mg 3 times/day (450 mg)

–*CHF:* PO: 12.5 mg 2–3 times/day given with a diuretic and a digitalis, and/or cardiac glycoside preparation, increasing up to 50 mg 2–3 times/day if needed

PEDIATRIC

–Safe use in children not established

ADVERSE/SIDE EFFECTS

RAPID

–Hypotension
–Bradycardia
–Bronchospasm
–Acute reversible renal failure
–Rash
–Angioedema
–Shortness of breath/dyspnea/cough
–Fever/chills

GRADUAL

–Impotence
–Dysuria
–Nocturia
–Proteinuria
–Nephrotic syndrome
–Urinary frequency
–Neutropenia
–Hyperkalemia
–Loss of taste
–Dizziness/light-headedness
–Fatigue

CONTRAINDICATIONS

–Hypersensitivity
–Pregnant or lactating patients
–Heart block
–In conjunction with potassium-sparing diuretics
–Children

SPECIAL PRECAUTIONS

–Renal disease
–Thyroid disease
–COPD
–Asthma
–Dialysis patients
–Hypovolemia
–Hyperkalemia
–Leukemia

–Lupus erythematosus
–Diabetes mellitus

OTHER SPECIAL INFORMATION
–PO onset = 15–60 min; peak = 1–1½ hr; duration = 6 hr.
–Use with extreme caution in renal dysfunction.
–Do not give with potassium supplements.
–This drug is most effective when given with a diuretic.
–This drug should not be used with vasodilators or with potassium-sparing diuretics.
–Monitor BP frequently for decreases during use.
–Full therapeutic effects occur in approximately 2 weeks.

ANTIDOTE

SEVERE REACTIONS
–D/C drug immediately and initiate appropriate treatment for symptoms.
–Lavage stomach.
–Expand fluid volume with NS and place patient in supine, or Trendelenburg position for severe hypotension.
–Treat bradycardia with IV ATROPINE.
–Treat bronchospasm with IV THEOPHYLLINE and OXYGEN.
–Treat cardiac failure with diuretics.
–Treat severe reactions with hemodialysis.

OTHER REACTIONS
–Notify physician of any side effects and initiate appropriate actions.

CEFACLOR Ceclor

CLASS
–Antibiotic, 2nd-generation CEPHALOSPORIN

USES
–Otitis media
–Respiratory tract infections

–Skin infections
–Bone and joint infections
–Urinary tract infections
–Gynecological infections
–Septicemia

ACTION
–Inhibits cell wall synthesis

USUAL DOSAGE/ROUTE
ADULT
–PO: 250–500 mg every 8 hr (max dose 4 gm/day)
PEDIATRIC
–PO: 20–40 mg/kg/day every 8 hr in divided doses

ADVERSE/SIDE EFFECTS
RAPID
–NVD
–Anaphylaxis
GRADUAL
–Rash
–Superinfection

CONTRAINDICATIONS
–Hypersensitivity to CEPHALOSPORINS, PENICILLINS
–Use in infants less than 1 month old

SPECIAL PRECAUTIONS
–Pregnant or lactating patients
–Renal impairment

OTHER SPECIAL INFORMATION
–Drug effect decreases if used with TETRACYCLINES, ERYTHROMYCINS.
–Drug toxicity increased if used with FUROSEMIDE, AMINOGLYCOSIDES, PROBENECID, VANCOMYCIN.
–Monitor renal status, potassium, and sodium levels.
–Administer with food if GI upset occurs.

ANTIDOTE

SEVERE REACTIONS

–D/C drug immediately and initiate appropriate treatment for symptoms.

–Treat anaphylaxis with EPINEPHRINE, AMINOPHYLLINE, O_2, IV corticosteroids, antihistamines, and ALS procedures as appropriate.

OTHER REACTIONS

–Notify physician of any side effects and initiate appropriate actions.

CEFAZOLIN SODIUM   Ancef, Kefzol

CLASS

–Antibiotics, 1st-generation CEPHALOSPORIN

USES

–Infections caused by gram-negative bacilli, and gram-positive organisms

–Skin infections

–Urinary tract infections

–Bone and joint infections

–Respiratory tract infections

–Intraabdominal and biliary tract infections

ACTION

–Inhibits cell wall synthesis

USUAL DOSAGE/ROUTE

ADULT

–IV: 0.5–2.0 gm every 6–8 hr

–IM: 0.5–2.0 gm every 6–8 hr

PEDIATRIC (older than 1 month)

–IV: 25–50 mg/kg/day every 6–8 hr in divided doses

–IM: 25–50 mg/kg/day every 6–8 hr in divided doses

ADVERSE/SIDE EFFECTS

RAPID

–Anaphylaxis

GRADUAL

–NVD
–Rash
–Phlebitis and pain at IV site

CONTRAINDICATIONS

–Hypersensitivity to CEPHALOSPORINS, PENICILLINS
–Infants less than 1 month old

SPECIAL PRECAUTIONS

–Pregnant or lactating patients
–Renal impairment

OTHER SPECIAL INFORMATION

–Monitor renal function.
–Dose may need to be reduced if creatinine clearance is less than 54 ml/min.
–Drug action is reduced if given with TETRACYCLINE, ERYTHROMYCIN.
–Toxicity increases when given with AMINOGLYCOSIDES, FUROSEMIDE, PROBENECID.
–Not compatible in IV fluid containing TETRACYCLINE, ERYTHROMYCIN, calcium salts, magnesium salts, barbiturates, or aminoglycosides.
–Monitor IV site for irritation, extravasation.

ANTIDOTE

SEVERE REACTIONS

–D/C drug immediately and initiate appropriate treatment for symptoms.
–Treat anaphylaxis with EPINEPHRINE, AMINOPHYLLINE, O_2, IV corticosteroids, antihistamines, and ALS procedures as appropriate.

OTHER REACTIONS

–Notify physician of any side effects and initiate appropriate actions.

CEFTRIAXONE SODIUM Rocephin

CLASS
–Broad-spectrum antibiotic, 3d-generation CEPHALOSPORIN

USES
–Gram-negative and gram-positive organisms
–Lower respiratory tract infections
–Urinary tract infections
–Skin, bone and joint, and intraabdominal infections
–Septicemia
–Meningitis
–Gonorrhea

ACTION
–Inhibits cell wall synthesis

USUAL DOSAGE/ROUTE

ADULT
–IM: 1–2 gm/day in single dose or divided doses every 12 hr
–IV: 1–2 gm/day in single dose or divided doses every 12 hr; infuse over 30–60 min

PEDIATRIC
–IM: 50–75 mg/kg/day every 12 hr in divided doses
–IV: 50–75 mg/kg/day every 12 hr in divided doses

ADVERSE/SIDE EFFECTS

RAPID
–Anaphylaxis

GRADUAL
–NVD
–Anorexia
–Renal failure
–Thrombocytopenia

–Rash
–Phlebitis and pain at IM site

CONTRAINDICATIONS
–Hypersensitivity to CEPHALOSPORINS, PENICILLINS
–Infants less than 1 month old

SPECIAL PRECAUTIONS
–Pregnant or lactating patients
–Renal disease

OTHER SPECIAL INFORMATION
–Monitor prothrombin time (PT).
–Monitor renal function.
–Inject deep IM and massage.
–Drug effect is reduced if given with TETRACYCLINES, ERYTHROMYCIN.
–Drug toxicity increases if given with AMINOGLYCOSIDES, FUROSEMIDES, PROBENECID.

ANTIDOTE
SEVERE REACTIONS
–D/C drug immediately and initiate appropriate treatment for symptoms.
–Treat anaphylaxis with EPINEPHRINE, AMINOPHYLLINE, O_2, IV corticosteroids, antihistamines, and ALS procedures as appropriate.
OTHER REACTIONS
–Notify physician of any side effects and initiate appropriate actions.

CEPHALOTHIN SODIUM Ceporacin, Keflin, Seffin

CLASS
–Broad-spectrum antibiotic, 1st-generation CEPHALOSPORIN

USES
–Gram-negative bacilli and gram-positive organisms
–Infections of skin, urinary tract, bone and joint, lower respiratory tract
–Endocarditis, septicemia
–Bacterial peritonitis

ACTION
–Inhibits cell wall synthesis

USUAL DOSAGE/ROUTE
ADULT
–IM: 1–2 gm in divided doses every 4–6 hr
–IV: 1–2 gm in divided doses every 4–6 hr (not commonly administered in IV form)

PEDIATRIC
–IM: 80–160 mg/kg/day in divided doses every 6 hr
–IV: 80–160 mg/kg/day in divided doses every 6 hr

ADVERSE/SIDE EFFECTS
RAPID
–Anaphylaxis

GRADUAL
–NVD
–Rash
–Phlebitis and pain at injection site

CONTRAINDICATIONS
–Hypersensitivity to CEPHALOSPORINS, PENICILLINS

SPECIAL PRECAUTIONS
–Pregnant or lactating patients
–Renal impairment
–Patients over age 50

OTHER SPECIAL INFORMATION
–Inject deep IM and massage.
–Monitor IV site for phlebitis, change IV site every 48 hr.

–Administer direct IV 1 gm/10 ml solution slowly in 3–5 min.
–Intermittent infusion 1–2 gm in 50 ml solution administered over 15–30 min

ANTIDOTE

SEVERE REACTIONS

–D/C drug immediately and initiate appropriate treatment for symptoms.
–Treat anaphylaxis with EPINEPHRINE, AMINOPHYLLINE, O_2, IV corticosteroids, antihistamines, and ALS procedures as appropriate.

OTHER REACTIONS

–Notify physician of any side effects and initiate appropriate actions.

CHARCOAL, PURIFIED ORGANIC-ACTIVATED, USP Activated Charcoal, Charcoaide, Charcoal Powder, Charcocaps, Charcodote, Charcotabs, Digestalin, and others

CLASS

–Antidote, adsorbent, antiflatulent

USES

–To treat poisoning and flatulence
–To function as a deodorant in wounds
–To treat diarrhea
–Dyspepsia

ACTION

–Effectively absorbs wide variety of drugs and chemicals; not absorbed or metabolized by the body, and is excreted with feces
–Increases absorption in GI tract

USUAL DOSAGE/ROUTE

ADULT AND PEDIATRIC

–5–10 times the weight of poisonous substance ingested, using at least 30 g/250 ml water PO or NG tube
–PO: 500 mg–1 gm 3–4 times/day

ADVERSE/SIDE EFFECTS

RAPID

–N & V

GRADUAL

–Black stools
–Constipation

CONTRAINDICATIONS

–Hypersensitivity
–When given concurrently with other medication, can significantly reduce absorption of the drug
–Unconsciousness/semiconsciousness
–Cyanide poisoning
–Mineral acids poisoning
–Alkalies poisoning

SPECIAL PRECAUTIONS

–None known

OTHER SPECIAL INFORMATION

–Give after emesis; absorbs and inactivates syrup of ipecac.
–Powder form is most effective.
–Mix with tap water to make a thick syrup.
–Add flavoring or fruit juice to make more palatable.
–Do not mix with dairy products.
–Repeat dose if vomiting occurs soon after administered.

ANTIDOTE

SEVERE REACTIONS

–D/C drug immediately and initiate appropriate treatment for symptoms.

OTHER REACTIONS

–Notify physician of any side effects and initiate appropriate actions.

CHLORDIAZEPOXIDE HCL Libitabs, Librium, Sereen, Tenax, and others

CLASS

–Antianxiety agent, minor tranquilizer

USES

–Short-term treatment of anxiety, tension
–Management of acute alcoholism withdrawal symptoms
–Preoperative anxiety and apprehension

ACTION

–Depresses CNS brain stem reticular formation, limbic system, and polysynaptic reflex arcs in spinal cord
–Also may exhibit sedative, appetite stimulation, weak analgesia, and varying degrees of anticonvulsant activity

USUAL DOSAGE/ROUTE

ADULT

–PO: 5–25 mg 3–4 times/day
–IM, IV: 50–100 mg initially, followed by 25–50 mg 3–4 times/day
–*Preoperative*: 50–100 mg IM 1 hr before surgery

PEDIATRIC (over age 6)

–PO: 5 mg 2–4 times/day; may increase to 10 mg 2–3 times/day
–Not recommended in children under 6 years (use with caution in children under age 18)

ADVERSE/SIDE EFFECTS

RAPID

–N & V
–Dermatitis, itching

–Orthostatic hypotension
–Tachycardia
–Blurred vision

GRADUAL

–Drowsiness, ataxia, confusion (especially with geriatric and debilitated patients)
–Headache
–Agranulocytosis
–Tremors
–Fatigue
–Jaundice, hepatic dysfunction
–Insomnia
–Changes in EEG patterns
–Constipation

CONTRAINDICATIONS

–Hypersensitivity to drug
–Narrow-angle glaucoma
–Pregnancy
–Psychosis

SPECIAL PRECAUTIONS

–Elderly
–Liver disease
–Renal disease
–Debilitated patients

OTHER SPECIAL INFORMATION

–Overdosage is characterized by somnolence, confusion, coma, diminished reflexes, hypotension.
–Antidote: LEVOPHED or ARAMINE to combat hypotension and RITALIN or CAFFEINE to combat CNS depression.
–Administer PO drug with food or milk to lessen GI symptoms.
–Caution patients against combining the drug with alcohol.
–Caution in elderly due to long duration of action and accumulation of active metabolites.

ANTIDOTE

SEVERE REACTIONS

–D/C drug immediately; initiate appropriate treatment for symptoms.
–Treat hypotension with LEVOPHED or ARAMINE.
–Treat CNS depression with RITALIN or CAFFEINE.
–Lavage patient's stomach of any residual drug.

OTHER REACTIONS

–Notify physician of side effects; initiate appropriate actions.

CHLORPROMAZINE HCL, USP Clorazine, Ormazine, Promaz, Thorazine

CLASS

–Antipsychotic (major tranquilizer), antiemetic

USES

–Psychotic disorders
–Mental and emotional disturbances
–Intractable hiccups
–N & V
–Alcohol withdrawal
–Behavioral problems in children
–Migraine headache

ACTION

–Depression of the subcortical area of the brain and inhibition of the hypothalamus

USUAL DOSAGE/ROUTE

ADULT

–PO, IM, IV: 10–50 mg 3 times/day depending on condition being treated

PEDIATRIC

–PO, IM: 0.5 mg/kg 3–4 times daily

ADVERSE/SIDE EFFECTS

RAPID

–Laryngospasm
–Dyspnea
–Respiratory depression
–Dry mouth
–Tachycardia
–Hypotension
–Sedation
–N & V
–Cardiac arrest

GRADUAL

–Rash
–Headache
–Hepatotoxicity
–Leukopenias, agranulocytosis
–Extrapyramidal reactions
–Pseudoparkinsonism
–Constipation
–Anorexia
–Gynecomastia
–Orthostatic hypotension
–Urinary retention
–Menstrual irregularities

CONTRAINDICATIONS

–Hypersensitivity to phenothiazine derivatives
–Chronic alcoholism
–Barbiturate withdrawal states
–Bone marrow depression
–Liver damage
–History of glaucoma
–Cerebral arteriosclerosis

SPECIAL PRECAUTIONS

–Pregnant and lactating patients
–Seizure disorders
–Hypertensive disease

–Liver disease
Cardiac disease

OTHER SPECIAL INFORMATION
–Periodic blood checks are advised.
–Give IM slowly in upper outer quadrant of buttock; massage injection site well.
–Instruct patient that urine may be pink, red, or red-brown.
–Slight yellowing of parenteral preparation does not alter potency.

ANTIDOTE
SEVERE REACTIONS
–D/C drug immediately and initiate appropriate treatment for symptoms.
–Lavage patient's stomach for residual drug (do not induce vomiting).

OTHER REACTIONS
–Notify physician of any side effects and initiate appropriate actions.

CHLORPROPAMIDE Chloronase, Diabinese, Glucamide, Novopropamide, Stabinol

CLASS
–Oral hypoglycemic (1st-generation sulfonylurea antidiabetic)

USES
–For the treatment of stable maturity-onset noninsulin dependent diabetes mellitus (type II) uncontrolled by diet and exercise alone

ACTION
–Stimulates beta cells of pancreas to secrete insulin
–Increases receptor sites for insulin on cell walls
–Appears to inhibit glycogenolysis in the liver

USUAL DOSAGE/ROUTE

ADULT

–PO: 100–250 mg daily initially, then 100–500 mg daily maintenance according to response

PEDIATRIC

–Not for use in children

ADVERSE/SIDE EFFECTS

RAPID

–Hypoglycemia (tremors, pallor, diaphoresis, coma)
–Headache
–Weakness
–Erythema, urticaria

GRADUAL

–NVD
–Hypothyroidism incidence increases with duration of therapy
–CHF
–Hepatitis
–Aplastic anemia
–Hyponatremia

CONTRAINDICATIONS

–Hypersensitivity
–Brittle or juvenile diabetes
–Pregnancy
–Hepatic, renal, or thyroid dysfunction
–Diabetes mellitus adequately controlled by diet

SPECIAL PRECAUTIONS

–Elderly (requires reduced dosages)
–Thyroid disease
–Cardiac disease
–Renal disease
–Liver disease

OTHER SPECIAL INFORMATION

–Coumadin-type anticoagulants potentiate this drug.
–Dosage must be individualized.

–Use of alcohol concurrently may cause an Antibase type reaction (N & V, cramps, headache, hypoglycemia).
–Thiazide-type diuretics detract from the effectiveness of this drug.
–Assess patient for allergy to sulfa drugs.
–This drug may prolong action of barbiturates.
–Instruct patient to take this drug at the same time each day, and eat 30 minutes afterwards.
–Use cautiously in elderly patients; very long duration of activity.
–Drug onset = 1 hr; half-life = 36 hr; duration = 24–60 hr.

ANTIDOTE

SEVERE REACTIONS

–D/C drug immediately and initiate appropriate treatment for symptoms.
–Treat hypoglycemic reaction with 10–50% glucose solution IV.

OTHER REACTIONS

–Notify physician of any side effects and initiate appropriate actions.

CIMETIDINE HCL Tagamet

CLASS

–Histamine (H_2) receptor antagonist (antihistamine)

USES

–Accelerates healing of duodenal and gastric ulcers and pathological hypersecretory conditions (Zollinger–Ellison syndrome and multiple myelomas)

ACTION

–Inhibits histamine at the H_2 receptor site in parietal cells of the stomach, thus preventing secretion of gastric acid

USUAL DOSAGE/ROUTE

ADULT AND PEDIATRIC (over 16 years)

–PO: 300 mg 4 times daily with meals and at bedtime for 8 weeks, then give 300–400 mg at bedtime

–IV: 300 mg diluted in 20 ml NaCl injected over 1–2 min every 6 hr, or 300 mg/50 ml D_5W infused over 15–20 min every 6 hr not to exceed 2,400 mg/24 hr

PEDIATRIC (under 16 years)

–Not for use in children

ADVERSE/SIDE EFFECTS

RAPID

–Confusion, agitation
–Slurred speech
–Bradycardia
–Headache
–Convulsions
–Rash, urticaria

GRADUAL

–Transient maculopapular or acne-like rashes
–Mild and transient diarrhea
–Gynecomastia
–Jaundice
–Impotence
–Increase in BUN & creatinine
–Increase in bleeding time
–Aplastic anemia

CONTRAINDICATIONS

–Hypersensitivity

SPECIAL PRECAUTIONS

–Pregnant and lactating patients
–Organic brain syndrome
–Liver disease
–Renal disease

OTHER SPECIAL INFORMATION

–This drug may potentiate warfarin effect and increase bleeding time.
–Peak = 1–1 ½ hr; half-life = 1 ½ hr; duration 4–5 hr.
–Safe use in children under age 16 is not established.
–Antacids decrease absorption of this drug.

ANTIDOTE

SEVERE REACTIONS

–D/C drug immediately and initiate appropriate treatment for symptoms.

OTHER REACTIONS

–Notify physician of any side effects and initiate appropriate actions.

CIPROFLOXACIN HCL Cipro

CLASS

–Anti-infective (quinolone antibiotic)

USES

–Lower respiratory tract infections
–Severe urinary tract infections
–Skin and skin structure infections
–Infectious diarrhea
–Bone and joint infections

ACTION

–Inhibits bacterial DNA synthesis

USUAL DOSAGE/ROUTE

ADULT

–PO: 500–750 mg every 12 hr
–IV: 400 mg every 12 hr

PEDIATRIC

–Safe use in children not established

ADVERSE/SIDE EFFECTS

RAPID

–NVD
–Restlessness
–Seizures
–Rash

GRADUAL

–Chills, fever
–Headache
–Constipation
–Dizziness
–Abdominal pain
–Crystalluria
–Hematuria
–Photosensitivity
–Confusion
–Tremors
–Hallucinations
–Tinnitus
–Blurred vision

CONTRAINDICATIONS

–Hypersensitivity
–Pregnant or lactating patients
–Children
–Severe dehydration

SPECIAL PRECAUTIONS

–Renal disease
–Hepatic disease
–CNS disturbances
–Seizures
–Cerebral arteriosclerosis

OTHER SPECIAL INFORMATION

–Monitor urine output for decreases (patients must be well hydrated to use this drug).
–Monitor urine alkalinity to prevent crystalluria.
–This drug increases THEOPHYLLINE levels that may cause toxicity.

–Administer when patient's stomach is empty for best absorption.
–Antacids may reduce drug absorption.
–If needed, give antacids at least 2 hr before or after dosage of drug.
–Increased blood levels occur when used with PROBENECID.
–Effectiveness decreases with NITROFURANTOIN (MACRADONTIN).

ANTIDOTE

SEVERE REACTIONS
–D/C drug immediately and initiate appropriate treatment for symptoms.
–Treat PO overdose with lavage and maintain hydration.
–Hemodialysis or peritoneal dialysis

OTHER REACTIONS
–Notify physician of any side effects and initiate appropriate actions.

CLARITHROMYCIN Biaxin

CLASS
–Semisynthetic macrolide antibiotic

USES
–Mild-to-moderate infections in upper and lower respiratory tract conditions involving many gram-positive and gram-negative organisms
–Uncomplicated skin and skin structure infections due to staphylococcus aureus or streptococcus pyogenes

ACTION
–Exerts an antibacterial/antimicrobial action by binding to the 5OS ribosomal subunit of susceptible organisms, inhibiting protein synthesis

USUAL DOSAGE/ROUTE

ADULT

–PO: 250–500 mg every 12 hr for 7–14 days

PEDIATRIC

–Safety in children under age 12 has not been established.

ADVERSE/SIDE EFFECTS

RAPID

–NVD
–Rash/urticaria/pruritus

GRADUAL

–Pseudomembranous colitis
–Abnormal taste
–Dyspepsia/abdominal pain
–Headache
–Elevated BUN
–Hepatotoxicity
–Abdominal pain

CONTRAINDICATIONS

–Hypersensitivity to this drug, or ERYTHROMYCIN, or other macrolydes
–Pregnancy
–Severe renal disease
–Severe liver disease

SPECIAL PRECAUTIONS

–Lactating patients
–Liver disease
–Renal disease (requires reduced dosing)
–Older adults with renal impairment (requires reduced dosing)

OTHER SPECIAL INFORMATION

–PO onset = 2 hr; peak = 2–3 days.
–This drug may increase serum concentrations of THEOPHYLLINE when used concurrently.

–Concurrent use with DIGOXIN may elevate digoxin levels.
–This drug is not affected by administration with or without meals.

ANTIDOTE

SEVERE REACTIONS

–D/C drug immediately and initiate appropriate treatment for symptoms.
–Treat anaphylaxis with ALS protocols as appropriate, including OXYGEN, IV EPINEPHRINE, IV THEOPHYLLINE, IV corticosteroids.

OTHER REACTIONS

–Notify physician of any side effects and initiate appropriate actions.

CLINDAMYCIN HCL, CLINDAMYCIN PALMITATE HCL, CLINDAMYCIN PHOSPHATE Cleocin, Dalacin-C

CLASS

–Antibiotic, antibacterial macrolide

USES

–Penicillin-resistant gram-positive infections and in patients who are allergic to penicillin
–Anaerobic infections below the diaphragm

ACTION

–Semisynthetic bacteriostatic that inhibits ribosomal protein synthesis

USUAL DOSAGE/ROUTE

ADULT

–PO: 150–300 mg every 6 hr (average 150 mg every 6 hr)
–IM, IV: 300–600 mg every 6–12 hr, max 4,800 mg/24 hr

PEDIATRIC

–*Moderate infections:* PO: 8–12 mg/kg/day in 3–4 divided doses

–*Severe infections:* PO: 12–25 mg/kg/day in 3–4 divided doses

ADVERSE/SIDE EFFECTS

RAPID

–N & V
–Rash, urticaria
–Anaphylaxis
–Diarrhea

GRADUAL

–Transient leukopenia
–Pseudomembranous colitis
–Elevated SGOT, alkaline phosphatase, bilirubin
–Thrombocytopenia
–Vaginitis
–Urinary frequency
–Abcess at injection site

CONTRAINDICATIONS

–Known hypersensitivity to this drug or LINCOMYCIN
–History of GI disease, especially colitis

SPECIAL PRECAUTIONS

–Liver disease
–Renal disease
–Asthma
–Newborns
–Pregnant or lactating patients

OTHER SPECIAL INFORMATION

–Give IM dosages deep into a large muscle.
–Check IV site daily for irritation or phlebitis.
–Drug must be taken on an empty stomach with a full glass of water 1–2 hr before meals.
–Drug must be taken in equal intervals around the clock to maintain blood levels.
–Do not administer drug as an undiluted bolus IV.

ANTIDOTE

SEVERE REACTIONS

–D/C drug immediately and initiate appropriate treatment for symptoms.

–Treat anaphylaxis with EPINEPHRINE, AMINOPHYLLINE, OXYGEN, and IV corticosteroids. Endotracheal intubation may also be required.

OTHER REACTIONS

–Notify physician of any side effects and initiate appropriate actions.

CLONIDINE HCL Catapres, Catapres-TTS, Dixarit

CLASS

–Antihypertensive (alpha-adrenergic agonist)

USES

–Management of mild-to-moderate hypertension

–Prophylaxis of vascular headaches

–Adjunctive therapy in opiate withdrawal

–Treatment of menopausal syndrome

ACTION

–Decreases blood pressure, pulse rate, and cardiac output by stimulating alpha-adrenergic receptors to inhibit cardioacceleration and vasoconstriction

USUAL DOSAGE/ROUTE

ADULT

–PO: 0.1 mg 2 times/day initially, then maintenance dose of 0.2–1.2 mg/day in 2–3 divided doses

–Topically: 1–3 mg applied weekly as transdermal delivery system

PEDIATRIC

–Safe use in children not established

ADVERSE/SIDE EFFECTS

RAPID
–Hypotension
–Bradycardia
–Palpitations
–Rash
–Pruritus

GRADUAL
–Drowsiness
–Dry mouth
–Nightmares
–Nervousness
–Depression
–Impotence
–Contact dermatitis from transdermal patch
–Sodium retention/weight gain
–Withdrawal phenomenon
–Glucose intolerance

CONTRAINDICATIONS
–Hypersensitivity

SPECIAL PRECAUTIONS
–Pregnant or lactating patients
–Cardiac disease
–Diabetes mellitus
–Myocardial infarction
–Cerebrovascular disease
–Renal insufficiency
–History of depression
–Use with other antihypertensives

OTHER SPECIAL INFORMATION
–Do not discontinue use of this drug abruptly (may cause rebound hypertension).
–Dosage may need to be reduced in elderly.
–Sedation increases if used with CNS depressants such as alcohol, antihistamines, narcotics, sedatives/hypnotics.

- Hypotension increases if used with antihypertensives or nitrates.
- Bradycardia increases if used with myocardial depressants or beta-adrenergic blockers.
- Decreased antihypertension effect if used with MAO inhibitors or tricyclic antidepressants.
- Abrupt discontinuation of drug will cause withdrawal symptoms.
- Transdermal absorption is greatest on chest or upper arm.
- Rotate transdermal sites each week.
- PO should be taken at same time every day.
- This drug may also be used to treat nicotine withdrawal.

ANTIDOTE

SEVERE REACTIONS

- D/C drug immediately and initiate appropriate treatment for symptoms.
- Treat overdose with gastric lavage and administration of activated charcoal.
- Treat hypotension with IV DOPAMINE.
- Treat bradycardia with IV ATROPINE.
- Treat rebound hypertension with TULAZOLINE HCL.

OTHER REACTIONS

- Notify physician of any side effects and initiate appropriate actions.

COCAINE HCL Cocaine

CLASS

- Topical anesthetic

USES

- Local (topical) anesthetic for mucous membranes

ACTION

- Produces anesthesia by preventing initiation and transmission of nerve impulses at the cell membrane

USUAL DOSAGE/ROUTE

ADULT AND PEDIATRIC

–5–10% instillation into the nose or throat
–4% instillation into the eye

ADVERSE/SIDE EFFECTS

RAPID

–Nervousness
–Excitation
–Vasomotor collapse

GRADUAL

–Addiction with chronic use
–Cornea may become dry and damaged

CONTRAINDICATIONS

–History of hypersensitivity

OTHER SPECIAL INFORMATION

–Drug of abuse, high psychological addiction.
–Not to be applied to abrased mucous membranes
–Not for injection
–Store under lock and key
–Onset = 1–5 min; duration = ½–1 hr.
–Be alert for nasal bleeding after the effect of the drug is worn off.

ANTIDOTE

SEVERE REACTIONS

–D/C drug immediately and initiate appropriate treatment for symptoms.

OTHER REACTIONS

–Notify physician of any side effects and initiate appropriate actions.

CODEINE PHOSPHATE, CODEINE SULFATE Codeine

CLASS
–Narcotic analgesic (opiate)

USES
–Relief of moderate-to-severe pain
–Antitussive for nonproductive cough

ACTION
–Analgesic properties may be related to interference with pain impulses at the subcortical level of the brain.

USUAL DOSAGE/ROUTE

ADULT
–PO, SQ, IM: Usual dose is 15–60 mg every 4 hr as needed
–*Antitussive:* 8–20 mg every 4–6 hr, max 120 mg/day

PEDIATRIC
–PO, SQ, IM: 3 mg/kg/day individual doses every 4–6 hr as needed
–*Antitussive:* 1–1.5 mg/kg/24 hr or 33–50 mg/M^2/24 hr divided in 3–4 doses not to exceed 60 mg/day

ADVERSE/SIDE EFFECTS

RAPID
–Drowsiness
–Sedation
–Dizziness
–Respiratory depression
–Lethargy
–N & V
–Bradycardia/tachycardia
–Palpitations
–Orthostatic hypotension
–Flushing, rash, urticaria

GRADUAL

–Gastric upset
–Constipation
–Anorexia
–Urinary retention

CONTRAINDICATIONS

–Hypersensitivity to opiates or any of the combination ingredients (ASA, ACETAMINOPHEN, CAFFEINE, PHENACETIN)
–Respiratory depression or severe disorders
–Increased intracranial pressure
–Seizure disorders

SPECIAL PRECAUTIONS

–Elderly
–Cardiac dysrhythmias
–Pregnant or lactating patients
–Head trauma
–Severe pulmonary disease

OTHER SPECIAL INFORMATION

–If nausea occurs, have patient lie down in darkened room to decrease vestibular stimulation and nausea.
–Administer with meals to diminish gastric upset.
–Concurrent use of alcohol or other CNS depressants increases the effects of the drug.
–Keep under lock and key (controlled substance).
–Drug may be habit-forming with chronic use.
–Onset = 15–30 min; peak = 1–2 hr; half-life = 2 ½–4 hr; duration = 4–6 hr.

Combination tablets are labeled as follows:

#1 = ¼ grain (15 mg) codeine
#2 = ½ grain (30 mg) codeine
#3 = ¾ grain (45 mg) codeine
#4 = 1 grain (60 mg) codeine

ANTIDOTE

SEVERE REACTIONS

–D/C drug immediately and initiate appropriate treatment for symptoms.

–Treat respiratory depression with OXYGEN.

–Treat overdose with NALOXONE as an antidote.

OTHER REACTIONS

–Notify physician of any side effects and initiate appropriate actions.

CORTISONE ACETATE Cortistan, Cortogen, Cortone

CLASS

–Corticosteroid synthetic

USES

–Inflammation

–Severe allergy

–Adrenal insufficiency

ACTION

–Inhibits the release of proteolytic enzymes by stabilizing the cell membrane, thus preventing the normal inflammatory response

–Decreases the number of lymphocytes, plasma cells, and eosinophils in the blood, thus interfering with the immune and allergic response

USUAL DOSAGE/ROUTE

ADULT AND PEDIATRIC

–PO: 25–300 mg daily but must be individualized according to patient response

–IM: 5–300 mg daily but must be individualized according to patient response

ADVERSE/SIDE EFFECTS

RAPID

–Circulatory collapse
–Tachycardia
–NVD

GRADUAL

–Fluid and electrolyte imbalance (potassium loss; retention of sodium and water)
–Cushing's syndrome
–Gastric or duodenal ulcers
–Acne
–Poor wound healing
–Psychoses
–Depression
–Menstrual abnormalities
–Headache
–Thrombophlebitis
–Embolism
–CHF
–GI hemorrhage
–Increased appetite
–Decreased growth in children
–Edema
–Moon face, buffalo hump

CONTRAINDICATIONS

–History of hypersensitivity
–Hypokalemia
–Systemic fungal infections

SPECIAL PRECAUTIONS

–Diabetes (can cause hyperglycemia)

OTHER SPECIAL INFORMATION

–Administer oral preparations with meals to minimize gastric upset.
–Monitor serum potassium.
–The drug causes immunosuppression and may mask symptoms of infection.

–Gradually decrease dosage after long-term therapy (adrenal crisis can occur if abruptly stopped).
–Patient may need a salt-restricted diet and potassium supplements.

ANTIDOTE

SEVERE REACTIONS

–D/C drug immediately and initiate appropriate treatment for symptoms.
–Observe and treat patient for hypotensive episode from adrenal crisis reaction.

OTHER REACTIONS

–Notify physician of any side effects and initiate appropriate actions.

DEFEROXAMINE MESYLATE Desferal

CLASS
–Heavy metal antagonist/antidote (chelating agent)

USES
–Acute, chronic iron intoxication
–Secondary iron overload associated with multiple transfusions

ACTION
–Removes excess iron by chelating unbound iron making a water-soluble complex that can be excreted by the kidneys

USUAL DOSAGE/ROUTE
ADULT
–IM or IV: 1 gram initially, then 500 mg every 4 hr for 2 doses, then 500 mg every 4–12 hr not to exceed 6 grams/day (IV rate should not exceed 15 mg/kg hourly).

PEDIATRIC (over 3 years)
–IM or IV: 1 gram initially, then 500 mg every 4 hr for 2 doses, then 500 mg every 4–12 hr not to exceed 6 grams/day or 20 mg/kg

ADVERSE/SIDE EFFECTS
RAPID
–Anaphylaxis
–Hypotension
–Tachycardia
–Pain at injection site
–Urticaria
–Blurred vision
–Abdominal cramps

GRADUAL
–Diarrhea
–Dysuria

–Optic neuropathy
–Audiographic hearing loss
–Red urine
–Erythema
–Leg cramps
–Fever

CONTRAINDICATIONS
–Hypersensitivity
–Pregnancy
–Severe renal disease
–Anuria
–Children under age 3

SPECIAL PRECAUTIONS
–Pregnant or lactating patients
–Pylonephritis
–Existing hearing defects
–Existing vision defects
–Elderly

OTHER SPECIAL INFORMATION
–Rapid IV infusion causes more side effects.
–This drug may be administered at the same time as blood.
–Ascorbic acid given with this drug may increase effectiveness of ascorbic acid and increase cardiac iron toxicity.

ANTIDOTE

SEVERE REACTIONS
–D/C drug immediately and initiate appropriate treatment for symptoms.
–ALS procedures, as appropriate, may include EPINEPHRINE, AMINOPHYLLINE, OXYGEN, IV corticosteroids, and antihistamines.
–Hemodialysis

OTHER REACTIONS
–Notify physician of any side effects and initiate appropriate actions.

DEXAMETHASONE, DEXAMETHASONE ACETATE, DEXAMETHASONE SODIUM PHOSPHATE Decadron, Deronil, Dexameth, and others

CLASS

–Long-acting corticosteroid (glucocorticoid)

USES

–Inflammation
–Endocrine disorders
–Rheumatic diseases
–Collagen diseases
–Dermatologic diseases
–Allergic states
–Ophthalmologic diseases
–Respiratory diseases
–Hematologic disorders
–Neoplastic diseases
–Cerebral edema secondary to tumor, cranial surgery, head trauma
–Septic shock
–Spinal cord trauma

ACTION

–Suppresses inflammation and the normal immune response

USUAL DOSAGE/ROUTE

ADULT

–PO: 0.75–9.0 mg in 2–4 divided doses

ACETATE

–IM: 8–16 mg at 1–3 week intervals
–Intraarticular: 4–16 mg at 1–3 week intervals
–Intralesional: 0.8–1.6 mg at 1–3 week intervals

SODIUM PHOSPHATE

–IV: 0.5–36 mg/day
 IM: 0.5–36 mg/day

–Intraarticular and intralesional: 0.5–36 mg/day

ADULT SHOCK

–IV: 40 mg every 4–6 hr or 20 mg IV loading dose with 3 mg/kg/24 hr continuous infusion

CEREBRAL EDEMA (bleeding, tumor, trauma)

–10–20 mg IV, then 4–10 mg IV, IM every 6 hr

PEDIATRIC

–PO: 24–340 mcg/kg/24 hr in divided doses or 660 mcg–10 mg/M^2/24 hr in 4 divided doses

SODIUM PHOSPHATE

–IV, IM, intraarticular, intralesional: 6–40 mcg/kg 1–2 times daily

ADVERSE/SIDE EFFECTS

RAPID

–Anaphylaxis
–PVCs
–Restlessness

GRADUAL

–Psychosis
–Gastric ulceration
–Depression
–Euphoria
–Increased intracranial pressure (children)
–Muscle wasting
–Reactivation of latent tuberculosis
–Hyperglycemia
–Increased intraocular pressure
–Hypertension
–N & V
–Adrenal suppression
–Edema
–Moon face, buffalo hump
–Decreased wound healing
–Osteoporosis

CONTRAINDICATIONS

–Hypersensitivity
–Systemic fungal infections

SPECIAL PRECAUTIONS

–Pregnant or lactating patients
–Chronic treatment may lead to adrenal suppression
–Children
–Diabetes mellitus
–Glaucoma
–Osteoporosis
–Ulcerative colitis
–Seizure disorders

OTHER SPECIAL INFORMATION

–Dosage should be increased for a short time after surgery or unusual stress.
–This drug is more potent than CORTISONE ACETATE.
–Drug lacks the sodium-retaining property of most steroids.
–Administer PO drug with meals to diminish gastric upset.
–This drug may mask symptoms of infection.
–Not recommended as replacement therapy in adrenal cortical insufficiency.
–Never abruptly discontinue.
–Do not use in alternate day therapy.
–Use lowest possible dose for shortest period of time.

ANTIDOTE

SEVERE REACTIONS

–D/C drug immediately and initiate appropriate treatment for symptoms.
–Observe and treat patient for hypotensive episode from adrenal crisis reaction

OTHER REACTIONS

–Notify physician of any side effects and initiate appropriate actions.

DEXAMETHASONE 0.1%-NEOMYCIN-BACITRACIN-POLYMYXIN B SULFATE COMBINATION Maxidex, Maxitrol, Neosporin, Otobiotic, Polymyxin B, Polysporin, Pyocidin, and others

CLASS

–Antibiotic combination with a corticosteroid

USES

–Treatment of ocular inflammation when concurrent use of an antimicrobial is necessary

ACTION

–Suppresses inflammatory response while having antimicrobial response through ingredients neomycin sulfate and polymyxin B sulfate to reduce such organisms as staphylococcus aureus, streptococcus viridans, Escherichia coli, klebsiella pneumonias, proteus, hemophilus influenzas, pseudomonas, aerobacter aerogenes, and Koch–Weeks bacillus

USUAL DOSAGE/ROUTE

ADULT AND PEDIATRIC

–Suspension: 1–2 drops topically in the conjunctival sac 4–6 times daily
–Ointment: A small amount into the conjunctival sac up to 3–4 times daily, or may be used adjunctively with drops at bedtime; not more than 20 ml or 8 gm should be used initially
–Skin cream: Apply lightly to affected area as needed
–GU irrigant: 1 ml/1000 cc NS continuous irrigation

ADVERSE/SIDE EFFECTS

RAPID

–Headache
–Restlessness

GRADUAL

–Elevation of intraocular pressure with possible development of glaucoma and optic nerve damage
–Posterior subcapsular cataract formation
–Delayed wound healing
–Secondary infection
–Local skin reactions, especially when applied to mucous membranes

CONTRAINDICATIONS

–Hypersensitivity to drug
–Epithelial herpes simplex
–Varicella of cornea and conjunctiva
–Mycobacterial infection of the eye
–After uncomplicated removal of a corneal foreign body

OTHER SPECIAL INFORMATION

–Educate patient regarding proper method of administering eye drops and eye ointment.
–Monitor for secondary infection.

ANTIDOTE

SEVERE REACTIONS

–D/C drug immediately and initiate appropriate treatment for symptoms.

OTHER REACTIONS

–Notify physician of any side effects and initiate appropriate actions.

DEXTROSE 50% Glucose, Insta-glucose

CLASS

–Carbohydrate caloric agent

USES

–Hypoglycemia

ACTION

–Provides carbohydrate calories to increase caloric intake in prevention and treatment of hypoglycemia

USUAL DOSAGE/ROUTE

ADULT

–IV: Individualized, severe hypoglycemia: 50–100 ml of 50% over 1 min

PEDIATRIC

–IV: 250–500 mg/kg of 25%

ADVERSE/SIDE EFFECTS

RAPID

–CHF
–Pulmonary edema
–Hyperglycemia

GRADUAL

–Hypertension
–Confusion
–Glycosuria
–Rebound hypoglycemia
–Extravasation necrosis

CONTRAINDICATIONS

–Hypersensitivity
–Hyperglycemia
–Delirium tremens
–Cranial or spinal hemorrhage
–CHF

SPECIAL PRECAUTIONS

–Renal disease
–Liver disease
–Cardiac disease
–Diabetes mellitus

OTHER SPECIAL INFORMATION

–Monitor IV site for extravasation.
–Monitor blood sugar frequently during and after use.

ANTIDOTE

SEVERE REACTIONS

–D/C drug immediately and initiate appropriate treatment for symptoms.

OTHER REACTIONS

–Notify physician of any side effects and initiate appropriate actions.

DIAZEPAM Valium

CLASS

–Antianxiety agent

USES

–Anxiety
–Alcohol withdrawal
–Seizure disorders
–Tetanic muscle spasms

ACTION

–Depresses subcortical limbic system, reticular formation

USUAL DOSAGE/ROUTE

ADULT

–PO: 2–10 mg 3–4 times/day
–PO extended release: 15–30 mg every day
–IV: 5–20 mg at 2 mg/min; may repeat every 5–10 min, not to exceed 60 mg; may repeat in 30 min

PEDIATRIC

–PO: 1.0–2.5 mg 3–4 times/day
–IV bolus: 0.1–0.3 mg/kg; repeat every 15 min × 2 doses; give at a rate of 1 mg/min over 3 min
–IM, IV: (child more than 5 yr): 5–10 mg every 3–4 hr as needed
–IM, IV: (infant more than 30 days): 1–2 mg every 3–4 hr as needed

ADVERSE/SIDE EFFECTS

RAPID

–Dizziness
–Orthostatic hypotension
–Tachycardia
–Blurred vision
–Respiratory depression

GRADUAL

–N & V
–Confusion
–Hallucinations
–Rash
–Tinnitus
–Constipation
–Dry mouth

CONTRAINDICATIONS

–Hypersensitivity
–Narrow-angle glaucoma
–Psychosis
–Pregnancy

SPECIAL PRECAUTIONS

–Debilitated patients and elderly
–Renal disease
–Hepatic disease

OTHER SPECIAL INFORMATION

–Drug action decreases with oral contraceptives, RIFAMPIN.
–Drug action increases with alcohol, CNS depressants.
–Give po with food or milk to prevent GI upset.
–IV and IM use of this drug is not compatible with other drugs and cannot be mixed.
–Give IV in large vein to reduce chance of extravasation.
–Take safety precautions to prevent injuries from drowsiness, dizziness.
–Avoid driving.
–Monitor liver studies.
–Avoid alcohol use when taking drug.

ANTIDOTE

SEVERE REACTIONS

–D/C drug immediately and initiate appropriate treatment for symptoms.

–Gastric lavage for PO ingestion

OTHER REACTIONS

–Notify physician of any side effects and initiate appropriate actions.

DIAZOXIDE Gliburide, Hyperstat, Proglycem

CLASS

–Antihypertensive agent (vasodilator)

USES

–Emergency reduction of diastolic blood pressure in hypertensive crisis (malignant hypertension)

–Increase blood glucose levels in hyperinsulinism

ACTION

–Decreases blood pressure by relaxing smooth muscle in peripheral arterioles

–Increases cardiac output while coronary and cerebral blood flow are maintained

USUAL DOSAGE/ROUTE

ADULT AND PEDIATRIC

–IV bolus: 1–3 mg/kg rapidly (less than 30 sec) up to 150 mg in a single dose; may be repeated at 5–15 min intervals until desired response is achieved

ADVERSE/SIDE EFFECTS

RAPID

–Hypotension

–Tachycardia

–Hyperglycemia in diabetics
–Headache
–NVD
–Dry mouth
–Rash
–Dizziness
–Rales
–Dyspnea
–Orthopnea
–Pain at the IV injection site

GRADUAL
–Sodium and water retention
–Phlebitis
–Edema
–Confusion
–Blurred vision
–Thrombocytopenia

CONTRAINDICATIONS
–Hypersensitivity to drug, thiazides, or sulfonamides
–Not for use in treatment of compensatory hypertension
–Pheochromocytoma
–Dissecting aortic aneurysm

SPECIAL PRECAUTIONS
–Tachycardia
–Fluid & electrolyte imbalances
–Pregnant or lactating patients
–Impaired cerebral or cardiac circulation
–Children

OTHER SPECIAL INFORMATION
–Monitor blood pressure until stabilized.
–Have patient remain lying down until at least 30 min after injection.
–This drug may potentiate effects of anticoagulants.
–Monitor urine for glucosuria.
–Onset = 1–2 min; peak = 5 min; duration = 3–12 hr with rapid IV injection.

–Do not mix with any drug or solution in syringe.
–Some clinical trials have suggested using constant infusions of DIAZOXIDE.

ANTIDOTE

SEVERE REACTIONS

–D/C drug immediately and initiate appropriate treatment for symptoms.
–Treat hypotension with LEVARTERENOL, DOPAMINE, or NOREPINEPHRINE, dialysis.
–Treat reflex tachycardia with a beta-blocker such as ESMOLOL.

OTHER REACTIONS

–Notify physician of any side effects and initiate appropriate actions.

DIGOXIN Lanoxicaps, Lanoxin

CLASS

–Cardiac glycoside (antidysrhythmic)

USES

–Congestive heart failure
–Atrial fibrillation and flutter
–Paroxysmal atrial tachycardia

ACTION

–Increases myocardial contraction efficiency by increasing influx of calcium ions into cells
–Increases cardiac output
–Slows the heart rate and increases vagal tone

USUAL DOSAGE/ROUTE

ADULT

–Loading dose: IV: 0.5 mg over 5 mins, then PO 0.125–0.5 mg/day every 4–6 hr
–Elderly PO: 0.125 mg every day maintenance

PEDIATRIC (1 month to 2 yr)
- –Loading dose: IV: 30–50 mcg/kg
- –Maintenance dose: 25–35% of loading dose daily divided every 12 hr

PEDIATRIC (2–5 yr)
- –Loading dose: IV: 25–35 mcg/kg
- –Maintenance: 25–35% of loading dose daily divided every 12 hr

PEDIATRIC (5–10 yr)
- –Loading dose: IV: 15–30 mcg/kg
- –Maintenance: 25–35% of loading dose daily divided every 12 hr

NEONATES (under 1 month)
- –Loading dose: IV: 25–30 mcg/kg
- –Maintenance dose: 25–35% of loading dose daily divided every 12 hr

PREMATURE INFANTS
- –Loading dose: IV: 0.04 mg/kg divided into 3 doses over 24 hr
- –Maintenance dose: IV: 0.01–0.03 mg/kg daily divided every 12 hr

ADVERSE/SIDE EFFECTS

RAPID
- –Dysrhythmias
- –Hypotension
- –AV block
- –Bradycardia

GRADUAL
- –Anorexia
- –NVD
- –Fatigue
- –Headache
- –Mental disturbances
- –Visual disturbances
- –Anorexia
- –Blurred vision
- –Yellow–green halos

CONTRAINDICATIONS
–Hypersensitivity to the drug
–Ventricular fibrillation
–Ventricular tachycardia
–Apical pulse less than 50
–Hypokalemia
–Carotid sinus syndrome

SPECIAL PRECAUTIONS
–Renal disease
–Acute MI, AV block
–Severe respiratory disease
–Hypothyroidism
–Elderly
–Pregnant or lactating patients

OTHER SPECIAL INFORMATION
–Digitoxin is a comparable preparation, yet its half-life is 5–7 days as opposed to digoxin with a half-life of 3 days.
–Correct hypokalemia prior to digoxin administration.
–Take apical pulse for 1 full min prior to giving drug; hold if pulse less than 60 and contact physician.
–Dose must be decreased in the elderly and in the presence of hepatic or renal dysfunction.
–Monitor drug levels in blood periodically (therapeutic level = 0.5–2.0 mg/ml).
–Do not administer calcium salts to digitalized patient.
–Administer IV slowly.
–After myocardial infarction, dilute with D_5W and give IV over 20–30 min.

ANTIDOTE

SEVERE REACTIONS
–D/C drug immediately and initiate appropriate treatment for symptoms.
–Treat hypokalemia with POTASSIUM.
–Monitor EKG for dysrhythmias.
–Treat hypotension with adrenergic blocking agents such as DOPAMINE

–Treat bradycardia with adrenergic blocking agents such as EPINEPHRINE HCL or ISOPROTERENOL HCL.

OTHER REACTIONS

–Notify physician of any side effects and initiate appropriate actions.

DIHYDROERGOTAMINE MESYLATE (D.H.E. 45)

CLASS

–Alpha-adrenergic blocker

USES

–Prophylaxis and treatment of vascular or migraine headaches

ACTION

–Direct stimulation of smooth muscle of peripheral and cranial vessels causing vasoconstriction.

USUAL DOSAGE/ROUTE

ADULT

–SQ, IM, IV: 1 mg and may repeat at 1–2-hr intervals for a total dose of 3 mg/24 hr with a maximum weekly dose of 6 mg

PEDIATRIC

–Safe use in children not established

ADVERSE/SIDE EFFECTS

RAPID

–None known

GRADUAL

–Transient tachycardia, bradycardia, precordial distress and pain, increased arterial pressure

–N & V

–Numbness, tingling, weakness in fingers, toes, and legs
–Muscle pain
–Localized edema and itching

CONTRAINDICATIONS
–Hypersensitivity
–Peripheral and occlusive vascular disease
–Coronary artery disease
–Hypertension
–Pregnancy
–Hepatic disease
–Renal disease
–Peptic ulcer
–Lactation
–Children

SPECIAL PRECAUTIONS
–None noted

OTHER SPECIAL INFORMATION
–Avoid prolonged administration; do not exceed recommended dose.
–This drug is most effective when administered at initial onset of headache.
–Provide quiet, low-light environment for patient to relax.
–Onset of action is 15–30 min after administration and persists for 3–4 hr.
–This drug resembles ERGOTAMINE but with less oxytoxic effects.

ANTIDOTE

SEVERE REACTIONS
–D/C drug immediately and initiate appropriate treatment for symptoms.
–Treat severe vasospasm with SODIUM NITROPRUSSIDE or TOLAZOLINE HCL and keep extremities warm.

OTHER REACTIONS
–Notify physician of any side effects and initiate appropriate actions.

DILTIAZEM HCL Cardizem, Cardizem SR

CLASS
–Calcium channel blocker

USES
–Chronic stable angina or vasospastic angina
–Coronary artery spasm
–Hypertension
–Atrial fibrillation/flutter (IV form)
–Paroxysmal superventricular tachycardia (IV form)

ACTION
–Inhibits calcium transport across the cell membrane during depolarization, thereby relaxing and dilating coronary and peripheral vascular smooth muscle

USUAL DOSAGE/ROUTE

ADULT
–PO: 30 mg 3–4 times/day increasing to a max of 360 mg/day
–IV: 0.25 mg/kg bolus over 2 min. If response is inadequate, repeat in 15 min using 0.35 mg/kg bolus over 2 min
–IV infusion: 5–15 mg/hr

PEDIATRIC
–Safe use in children not established

ADVERSE/SIDE EFFECTS

RAPID
–Dysrhythmias
–Bradycardia
–Hypotension
–Palpitations
–Heart block
–Angina
–NVD
–Rash

–Flushing
–Headache
–Itching and burning at IV injection site

GRADUAL
–Edema
–CHF
–Constipation
–Elevated liver function studies
–Acute renal failure
–Polyuria
–Fatigue
–Drowsiness
–Paresthesia

CONTRAINDICATIONS
–Hypersensitivity
–Sick sinus syndrome in the absence of a pacemaker
–2nd- or 3rd-degree heart block
–Cardiogenic shock
–Hypotension $<$ 90 mmHg systolic
–Acute MI
–Ventricular tachycardia
–Pulmonary congestion
–Atrial fibrillation or atrial flutter associated with Wolff–Parkinson–White syndrome, or short PR syndrome
–Inpatients who have recently received IV beta-blockers

SPECIAL PRECAUTIONS
–Pregnant or lactating patients
–CHF/PE
–Hypotension
–Acute liver injury
–Renal disease
–Children

OTHER SPECIAL INFORMATION
–Continuous IV infusion requires continuous ECG monitoring and frequent BP monitoring for hypotension.
–Onset of action of IV bolus is 3 min, and the duration of action is 1–3 hr, with a 95% response rate within 2–7 min.

–This drug causes increased effects of CIMETIDINE and DIGOXIN.
–Assess vital signs periodically during administration of this drug for decreases.
–This drug may cause a prolonged PR interval.

ANTIDOTE

SEVERE REACTIONS
–D/C drug immediately and initiate appropriate treatment for symptoms.
–Treat AV block with IV ATROPINE SULFATE.
–Treat hypotension with an IV vasopressor such as DOPAMINE.
–Implement ALS procedures as appropriate.

OTHER REACTIONS
–Notify physician of any side effects and initiate appropriate actions.

DIMENHYDRINATE Dimentabs, Dramamine, Reidamine, Vertibon, and others

CLASS
–Antiemetic, antihistamine (nonphenothiazine)

USES
–Prophylaxis and treatment of nausea, vomiting, and dizziness associated with motion sickness
–Ménière's disease
–Sedation

ACTION
–Acts centrally by blocking chemoreceptor trigger zone, which in turn acts on the vomiting center

USUAL DOSAGE/ROUTE

ADULT

–PO: 50–100 mg every 4 hr; IM, IR: 50 mg every 4 hours as needed; Rectally: 100 mg 1–2 times/day; or 50 mg IM, IV as needed

PEDIATRIC

–PO, IM, or Rectally: 6 mg/kg in divided doses 4 times/day not to exceed 300 mg daily

ADVERSE/SIDE EFFECTS

RAPID

–Palpitations
–Hypotension
–Blurred vision
–Convulsions in young children
–Rash, urticaria

GRADUAL

–Drowsiness
–Headache
–Dizziness
–Dry oral and respiratory passages

CONTRAINDICATIONS

–Hypersensitivity to narcotics
–Glaucoma
–Shock
–Pregnancy
–Lactation
–Cardiac or peripheral vascular disease
–Hypertension
–Seizures

SPECIAL PRECAUTIONS

–Elderly
–Children
–Cardiac dysrhythmias
–Asthma
–Prostatic hypertrophy

–Bladder neck obstruction
–Peptic ulcer

OTHER SPECIAL INFORMATION

–For IV infusion, dilute 50 mg in 10 ml of NS solution and infuse over 2 min.
–Caution patients against engaging in activities requiring alertness, such as driving or operating equipment.
–Undiluted solution may irritate and sclerose veins.
–This drug is ineffective for postoperative nausea and vomiting.

ANTIDOTE

SEVERE REACTIONS

–D/C drug immediately and initiate appropriate treatment for symptoms.

OTHER REACTIONS

–Notify physician of any side effects and initiate appropriate actions.

DIPHENHYDRAMINE HCL **Allerdryl, Baramine, Benadryl, Bendylate, Benylin, Compoz, Valdrene, Wehdryl, and others**

CLASS

–Antihistamine (H_1-receptor antagonist)

USES

–Allergic reactions
–Motion sickness
–Rhinitis
–Antiparkinsonism
–Sedation
–Prophylaxis to injection of certain drugs, such as X-ray dyes
–Infant colic

–Nonproductive cough
–Reversal of oculogyric crisis

ACTION

–Competes with histamine for H_1-receptor sites and thereby decreases allergic response
–Anticholinergic

USUAL DOSAGE/ROUTE

ADULT

–PO, IM, IV: 10–50 mg 3–4 times/day; maximum daily dose 400 mg
–*Anaphylaxis* or *phenothiazine idiosyncracy:* 10–50 mg deep IM or IV to maximum of 400 mg/24 hr

PEDIATRIC

–PO, IV, IM: 5 mg/kg/24 hr in 4 equally divided doses or 150 mg/M^2/24 hr in 4 equally divided doses to maximum of 300 mg/24 hr
–*Anaphylaxis* or *phenothiazine idiosyncracy:* 1.5 mg/kg IV bolus

ADVERSE/SIDE EFFECTS

RAPID

–Dizziness
–Drowsiness
–Vertigo
–Rash, urticaria
–Hypotension
–Palpitations
–Tachycardia

GRADUAL

–Fatigue
–Urinary retention
–Dryness of mouth, nose, throat
–Constipation
–Thickened mucous secretions from drying effect
–Thrombocytopenia

CONTRAINDICATIONS
–Hypersensitivity
–GI obstruction or stenosis
–Patient receiving MAO inhibitors (antidepressants)
–Asthma attacks
–Lower respiratory tract disease

SPECIAL PRECAUTIONS
–Increased intraocular pressure
–Renal disease
–Cardiac disease
–Hypertension
–Seizure disorder
–Stenosed peptic ulcers
–Hyperthyroidism
–Bladder neck obstruction
–Pregnant or lactating patients
–Prostatic hypertrophy

OTHER SPECIAL INFORMATION
–Give deep IM due to high incidence of muscle irritation.
–Increase dosing interval 1.5–2 times in moderate-to-severe renal failure.

ANTIDOTE

SEVERE REACTIONS
–D/C drug immediately and initiate appropriate treatment for symptoms.
–Treat overdose with IPECAC SYRUP or lavage, DIAZEPAM, vasopressors, short-acting barbiturates.

OTHER REACTIONS
–Notify physician of any side effects and initiate appropriate actions.

DISOPYRAMIDE PHOSPHATE DSP, Narpamide, Norpace, Norpaceor, Rythmodan

CLASS
–Antidysrhythmic (non-nitrate)

USES
–Unifocal and multifocal PVCs
–Premature ventricular contractions, paired (couplets)
–Episodes of ventricular tachycardia

ACTION
–Decreases rate of diastolic depolarization in cells with augmented automaticity and upstroke velocity while increasing the action potential duration of normal cardiac cells (similar to PROCAINAMIDE)

USUAL DOSAGE/ROUTE
ADULT (individualized)
–Loading dose PO: 300 mg then 150 mg every 6 hr
–Maintenance dose PO: 100–200 mg every 6 hr

ADULT (with small stature, renal or hepatic insufficiency)
–Loading dose: PO: 200 mg
–Maintenance dose: PO: 100 mg as determined by creatinine clearance rate

PEDIATRIC
–PO: 6–30 mg/kg/day in divided doses every 6 hr

ADVERSE/SIDE EFFECTS
RAPID
–Hypotension
–First-degree heart block
–Bradycardia
–Dry mouth, nose, throat, eyes (40%)
–Cardiac arrest
–Rash, urticaria

–Blurred vision
–Convulsions

GRADUAL
–Cardiac conduction disturbance
–Edema
–CHF
–Dizziness
–Headache
–Urinary retention (10–20%)
–Urinary frequency and urgency
–Constipation
–Hypoglycemia
–Thrombocytopenia

CONTRAINDICATIONS
–Hypersensitivity to drug
–Cardiogenic shock
–Preexisting 2nd- or 3rd-degree atrioventricular block (if no pacemaker is present)
–CHF
–Sick sinus syndrome
–Glaucoma
–Hypokalemia
–Urinary retention

SPECIAL PRECAUTIONS
–Pregnant or lactating patients
–Renal disease
–Diabetes mellitus
–Liver disease
–Myasthenia gravis
–Children
–Cardiomyopathy

OTHER SPECIAL INFORMATION
–Onset = 30 min; duration = 6–12 hr.
–This drug may be used in digitalized patients.
–Administer with caution to patients receiving other antidysrhythmic drugs.

–Monitor for adequate serum potassium levels.
–Drug does not have any alpha- or beta-adrenergic activity but does exhibit anticholinergic activity.
–Use with caution if a QT prolongation is greater than 25% of baseline.
–Patients in atrial fibrillation or flutter should be digitalized before drug use.

ANTIDOTE

SEVERE REACTIONS
–D/C drug immediately and initiate appropriate treatment for symptoms.
–Treat circulatory depression with DOPAMINE, OXYGEN, artificial ventilation, EKG.
–Treat convulsions with DIAZEPAM or THIOPENTAL.

OTHER REACTIONS
–Notify physician of any side effects and initiate appropriate actions.

DOBUTAMINE HCL Dobutrex

CLASS
–Synthetic adrenergic (catecholamine)

USES
–Indicated in the short-term treatment of refractory heart failure (cardiac decompensation)

ACTION
–Stimulates beta-1 (myocardial) adrenergic receptors to increase cardiac contractibility and cardiac output with minor effect on heart rate or peripheral blood vessels
–Increases renal and mesenteric perfusion

USUAL DOSAGE/ROUTE

ADULT

–IV: 2.5–10.0 mcg/kg/min and titrate to obtain desired hemodynamic and/or renal response up to 40 mcg/kg/min

PEDIATRIC

–Safe use in children not established

ADVERSE/SIDE EFFECTS

RAPID

–Angina
–Headache
–N & V
–Anxiety
–Dyspnea
–Hypertension
–Tachycardia
–PVCs

GRADUAL

–Heart burn
–Muscle cramps

CONTRAINDICATIONS

–Hypersensitivity
–Hypovolemia
–Idiopathic hypertrophic subaortic stenosis

SPECIAL PRECAUTIONS

–Pregnant or lactating patients
–Children
–Hypertension

OTHER SPECIAL INFORMATION

–Reconstitute in at least 50 ml of D_5W, NS, or LR.
–Formula for dosage calculation with microdrip factor only (60 gtt = 1 ml): weight in kg x 15 amount in mg to be mixed in 250 ml with this concentration, the number of drops per min is equal to the same number of mcg/kg/min.

Example: 15 gtt 1 min = 15 mcg/kg/min.
–Alkaline solutions inactivate DOBUTAMINE HCL.
–Intravenous solutions remain stable for 24 hr.
–Onset = 1–2 min; half-life = 2 min; peak = 10 min.
–Monitor hemodynamics constantly.
–This drug is often used with SODIUM NITROPRUSSIDE for additive effects.
–Administer cautiously to patients receiving beta-blocking drugs.
–Correct hypovolemia before administration.

ANTIDOTE

SEVERE REACTIONS
–D/C drug immediately and initiate appropriate treatment for symptoms.
–Treat hypertension with a beta-1 adrenergic blocker such as ATENOLOL.

OTHER REACTIONS
–Notify physician of any side effects and initiate appropriate actions.

DONNATAL Donnatal

CLASS
–Combination anticholinergic, antispasmodic

USES
–Adjunctive treatment of irritable bowel syndrome (spastic colon, mucous colitis, and acute enterocolitis)

ACTION
–Inhibits gastrointestinal smooth muscle contraction
–Delays gastric emptying time
–Inhibits secretion of gastric juices

USUAL DOSAGE/ROUTE

ADULT

–PO: 1–2 teaspoons liquid, 1–2 tablets, or 1–2 capsules 3–4 times daily

PEDIATRIC

–PO: 10 lb: 0.5–0.75 ml every 4–6 hr
20 lb: 1.25–2.0 ml every 4–6 hr
30 lb: 2.5 ml every 4–6 hr
50 lb: ¾–1 teaspoon every 4–6 hr
80 lb: 1–1½ teaspoon every 4–6 hr

ADVERSE/SIDE EFFECTS

RAPID

–Tachycardia
–Dizziness
–Drowsiness
–Excitement
–Agitation

GRADUAL

–Psychological dependence
–Blurred vision
–Increased ocular tension
–Weakness

CONTRAINDICATIONS

–Hypersensitivity
–Pregnant and lactating patients
–Glaucoma
–Gastrointestinal obstructive disease
–Unstable cardiovascular disease

SPECIAL PRECAUTIONS

–Elderly

OTHER SPECIAL INFORMATION

–This drug may decrease desired effects of anticoagulants requiring dosage adjustments.
–Until response is determined, caution patients against engaging in activities that require alertness, such as driving.

–Administer ½ hour before meals.
–This drug contains HYOSCYAMINE SULFATE 0.1037 mg, ATROPINE 0.0194 mg, HYOSCINE HBR 0.0065 mg, PHENOBARBITAL 16.2 mg.

ANTIDOTE

SEVERE REACTIONS

–D/C drug immediately and initiate appropriate treatment for symptoms.

OTHER REACTIONS

–Notify physician of any side effects and initiate appropriate actions.

DOPAMINE HCL Dopastat, Intropin, Revimine

CLASS

–Adrenergic (catecholamine) agent, vasopressor

USES

–Hypotension
–Poor perfusion
–Shock

ACTION

–Peripheral vasoconstriction (alpha-adrenergic stimulant)
–Central vasodilation (beta-adrenergic stimulant)
–Positive inotropic effects result in an increased cardiac output, renal blood flow, glomerular infiltration, and urine production, blood pressure

USUAL DOSAGE/ROUTE

ADULT

–IV infusion only: 2–10 mcg/kg/min up to 20 mcg/kg/min; rates up to 50 mcg/kg/min may be used with caution when titrating to patient's response

–Titrate to obtain desired hemodynamic and/or renal response.

PEDIATRIC

–IV infision only: 2–10 mcg/kg/min

ADVERSE/SIDE EFFECTS

RAPID

–Tachycardia
–Hypertension
–NVD
–Palpitations
–Angina
–Headache
–Dyspnea

GRADUAL

–Necrosis & tissue sloughing with extravasation
–Gangrene

CONTRAINDICATIONS

–Hypersensitivity
–Pheochromocytoma
–Ventricular fibrillation
–Uncorrected tachydysrhythmias

SPECIAL PRECAUTIONS

–Pregnant or lactating patients
–Embolism
–Peripheral vascular disease

OTHER SPECIAL INFORMATION

–Mix with D_5W and NS or a combination of dextrose and saline.
–Formula for dosage calculation with microdrip factor only (60 gtt/ml): weight in kg x 15 = amount in mg to be mixed in 250 ml; with this concentration, the number of drops per minute is equal to the same number of mcg/kg/min.
Example: 15 gtt/min = 15 mcg/kg/min.
–Alkaline solutions ($NAHCO_3$) inactivate the drug.
–This drug deteriorates after 24 hr.

–Taper the drug before cessation.
–Monitor hemodynamics constantly.
–Correct hypovolemia before administration.
–Do not use this drug within 2 weeks of the patient's taking MAO inhibitors for fear of hypertensive crisis.

ANTIDOTE

SEVERE REACTIONS

–D/C drug immediately and initiate appropriate treatment for symptoms.
–Treat hypertension with a beta-1 adrenergic blocker such as ATENOLOL.

OTHER REACTIONS

–Notify physician of any side effects and initiate appropriate actions.

DOXYCYCLINE CALCIUM, DOXYCYCLINE HYCLATE, DOXYCYCLINE MONOHYDRATE Doxy-C, Vibramycin, Vibra-Tabs, and others

CLASS

–Broad-spectrum antibiotic (tetracycline)

USES

–Infections caused by sensitive gram-negative and gram-positive organisms, trachoma, amebiasis, gonorrhea, or syphilis in patients allergic to penicillin

ACTION

–Exerts its effect by blocking the attachment of aminoacyl transfer RNA to ribosomes and thus interferes with protein synthesis

USUAL DOSAGE/ROUTE

ADULT

–PO, IM, IV: 200 mg every 12 hr first day, then 100 mg/day or 50–100 mg every 12 hr

PEDIATRIC (less than 46 kg)

–PO, IM, IV: 4.4 mg/kg/day in divided doses every 12 hr

ADVERSE/SIDE EFFECTS

RAPID

–Rash, urticaria
–Anaphylaxis

GRADUAL

–GI discomfort
–NVD
–Renal impairment
–Liver impairment
–Maculopapular and erythematous rashes
–Pseudomembranous colitis

CONTRAINDICATIONS

–Hypersensitivity to tetracyclines
–Renal impairment
–Children under age 8
–Pregnancy

SPECIAL PRECAUTIONS

–Liver disease
–Lactating patients

OTHER SPECIAL INFORMATION

–Permanent discoloration and inadequate calcification of teeth have been documented when used during last half of pregnancy and in children younger than age 8.
–Patient may take with milk if GI symptoms occur.
–Do not give with antacids.
–Do not infuse IV solutions more concentrated than 1 mg/ml.
–Especially appropriate to use in the elderly with reduced renal function.
–Peak = 1½–4 hr; half-life = 14–24 hr.

ANTIDOTE

SEVERE REACTIONS

–D/C drug immediately and initiate appropriate treatment for symptoms

OTHER REACTIONS

–Notify physician of any side effects and initiate appropriate actions.

ENALAPRIL MALEATE Vasotec

CLASS
–Angiotensin-converting enzyme (ACE) inhibitor (antihypertensive)

USES
–Hypertension

ACTION
–Inhibits angiotensin-converting enzyme conversion of angiotensin I to angiotensin II, decreasing arterial and venous vasoconstriction and reducing sodium retention

USUAL DOSAGE/ROUTE

ADULT
–PO: 5 mg/day, increasing to desired effect up to a max of 40 mg/day
–IV: 0.625–1.25 mg over 5 min every 6 hr

PEDIATRIC
–Safe use in children not established

ADVERSE/SIDE EFFECTS

RAPID
–Hypotension
–Tinnitus
–Bronchospasm
–Diplopia
–Rash
–Shortness of breath/dyspnea/cough
–Angioedema
–Fever/chills
–Chest pain
–Bradycardia
–Paresthesias
–NVD

GRADUAL
–Insomnia
–Dizziness/light-headedness
–Proteinuria
–Renal failure
–Neutropenia
–Agranulocytosis
–Urinary frequency
–Hyperkalemia
–Headache
–Colitis
–Loss of taste
–Alopecia
–Fatigue

CONTRAINDICATIONS
–Hypersensitivity
–Pregnant or lactating patients
–Heart block
–In conjunction with potassium-sparing diuretics
–Children

SPECIAL PRECAUTIONS
–Renal disease
–Thyroid disease
–COPD
–Asthma
–Dialysis patients
–Hypovolemia
–Hyperkalemia
–Diabetes mellitus

OTHER SPECIAL INFORMATION
–PO onset = 1 hr; IV onset = 15 min.
–Aspirin and antacids decrease the effects of this drug.
–Use with extreme caution in renal dysfunction.
–Do not give with potassium supplements, potassium-sparing diuretics or with vasodilators.
–Monitor BP frequently for decreases during use.
–This drug may cause proteinuria

–Dilute IV dose with 50 ml of a dextrose or saline solution and administer over 5 min.

ANTIDOTE

SEVERE REACTIONS

–D/C drug immediately and initiate appropriate treatment for symptoms.
–Lavage stomach for PO ingestion.
–Expand fluid volume with NS and place in supine or Trendelenburg position for severe hypotension.
–Treat bradycardia with IV ATROPINE.
–Treat bronchospasm with IV THEOPHYLLINE and OXYGEN.
–Treat cardiac failure with diuretics.
–Treat severe reactions with hemodialysis.

OTHER REACTIONS

–Notify physician of any side effects and initiate appropriate actions.

ENDAL–HD COMBINATION Endal–HD

CLASS

–Antitussive, decongestant, antihistamine

USES

–To control cough, relieve nasal congestion

ACTION

–Centrally acting antitussive activity plus antihistamine activity and reduction of nasal congestion

USUAL DOSAGE/ROUTE

ADULT

–PO: 2 tsp (10 ml) 3–4 times/day

PEDIATRIC

–PO (age 6–12): 1 tsp (5 ml) 3–4 times/day

ADVERSE/SIDE EFFECTS

RAPID

–Drowsiness
–Increased distress

GRADUAL

–Cardiac palpitations
–Nervousness
–Dizziness
–GI upset

CONTRAINDICATIONS

–Hypersensitivity to drug components
–Bronchial asthma
–Pulmonary emphysema
–Pregnancy
–Lactating mothers

SPECIAL PRECAUTIONS

–Diabetes
–Hyperthyroidism
–Hypertension
–Cardiovascular disease
–After thoracotomy or laparotomy

OTHER SPECIAL INFORMATION

–Each 30 ml of this drug is a combination of HYDROCODONE BITARTRATE 10 mg, PHENYLEPHRINE HCL 30 mg, and CHLORPHENIRAMINE MALEATE 12 mg.
–Before using for a cough, identify primary cause of cough.

ANTIDOTE

SEVERE REACTIONS

–D/C drug immediately and initiate appropriate treatment for symptoms

OTHER REACTIONS

–Notify physician of any side effects and initiate appropriate actions.

EPINEPHRINE BITARTRATE, EPINEPHRINE HCL, EPINEPHRINE HCL RACEMIC
Adrenalin Chloride, Sus-Phrine

CLASS
–Natural catecholamine, both alpha and beta properties

USES
–Ventricular fibrillation and asystole
–Poor cardiac compression and rhythm
–Anaphylaxis
–Reversible bronchospasm associated with bronchitis and emphysema
–Bronchial asthma
–Croup (viral tracheal bronchitis)

ACTION
–Alpha effects: peripheral vasoconstriction
–Beta effects: decreases bronchospasms by relaxing smooth muscles in bronchial tree and causes bronchial dilation
–Increases heart rate and cardiac output
–Increases atrioventricular conduction
–Increases cardiac irritability
–Increases myocardial contractile force
–Increases systemic vascular resistance
–Increases arterial blood pressure
–Increases myocardial oxygen consumption
–Increases automaticity
–Converts fine ventricular fibrillation to coarse ventricular fibrillation once acidosis is corrected

USUAL DOSAGE/ROUTES

ADULT (cardiac conditions)
–IV: 0.3–1.0 mg of 1:10,000 solution and may repeat at 5-min intervals
–Intracardiac or endotracheal tube: 0.3–1.0 mg of 1:10,000 solution. Each must be diluted in 10 ml of NS.

–SC: 0.1–0.3 ml of 1:200 solution (Sus-Phrine)
–PO inhalation: 1–2 puffs of 2.25% solution at 1–5-min intervals

ADULT (anaphylaxis, bronchospasm, hypersensitivity reactions)

–IV: 1.0–2.5 ml of 1:10,000 solution given slowly
–IM or SC: 0.1–0.5 ml of 1:1,000 solution and may repeat every 10–15 min 3 times

PEDIATRIC (cardiac conditions)

–IV or endotracheal tube: 0.01 mg/kg (or 10 mcg/kg) of 1:10,000 solution and may repeat at 5-min intervals
–SC: 0.005 ml/kg (Sus-Phrine)

PEDIATRIC (anaphylaxis, bronchospasm, hypersensitivity reactions)

–SC: 0.01–0.03 mg/kg of 1:1,000 solution and may repeat every 20 min up to 4 hr as needed

ADVERSE/SIDE EFFECTS

RAPID

–Increased heart rate
–Tachydysrhythmias
–Pallor, cool skin
–Tissue necrosis
–Nervousness, fear, anxiety, restlessness
–Tremors
–Dizziness, syncope
–N & V
–Throbbing headache
–Hypertension
–Altered state of perception and thought

GRADUAL

–Pulmonary edema
–Urinary retention
–Metabolic acidosis
–Elevated blood glucose

CONTRAINDICATIONS

–Hypersensitivity
–Cardiac asystole, electromechanical dissociation

–Narrow-angle glaucoma
–Hemorrhagic, traumatic, or cardiogenic shock
–Organic heart or brain disease
–Patients receiving CYCLOPROPANE, HALOTHANE, or Halogenated Hydrocarbon General Anesthetics because of increased cardiac irritability

SPECIAL PRECAUTIONS

–Prostatic hypertrophy
–Diabetes mellitus
–Hyperthyroidism
–Parkinson's disease
–Preexisting tachycardias, cardiovascular disease, hypertension
–Pregnancy (will decrease placental blood flow and may induce early labor)

OTHER SPECIAL INFORMATION

–In severe anaphylaxis, may give 0.1 mg of 1:1,000 solution SC at site of sting
–Must flush IV lines after use of $NaHCO_3$ or $CaCl_2$, (will precipitate)
–May widen patient's pulse pressure
–Repeated injections can cause tissue necrosis at the site of injection and in such organs as the kidneys and liver
–Must correct systemic metabolic acidosis for epinephrine to be nonionized and in the active form
–Rotate SC/IM sites, massage after injection.

ANTIDOTE

SEVERE REACTIONS

–D/C drug immediately and initiate appropriate treatment for symptoms.
–Treat toxicity shock with an antihypertensive agent such as NITROPRUSSIDE SODIUM.
–Treat cardiac dysrhythmias with a beta-adrenergic blocker such as PROPRANOLOL HCL.

OTHER REACTIONS

–Notify physician of any side effects and initiate appropriate actions.

ERYTHROMYCIN BASE, ERYTHROMYCIN ESTOLATE, ERYTHROMYCIN ETHYLSUCCINATE, ERYTHROMYCIN GLUCEPTATE, ERYTHROMYCIN LACTOBIONATE, ERYTHROMYCIN STEARATE **E.E.S., E-Mycin, Erythrocin, Robimycin, Wyamycin, and others**

CLASS

–Antibacterial (macrolide antibiotic)

USES

–The prevention and treatment of mild to moderately severe infections caused by sensitive group A betahemolytic streptococci, diplococcus pneumoniae, mycoplasma pneumoniae, corynebacterium diphtheriae, bordetella pertussis, listeria monocytogenes, neisseria gonorrheae, legionella pneumophila, etc.

ACTION

–Bacteriostatic action due to inhibition of ribosomal protein synthesis

USUAL DOSAGE/ROUTE

ADULT

–PO: 250–500 mg every 6 hr (base, estolate, stearate) or 400–800 mg every 6 hr (ETHYLSUCCINATE)
–IV: 15–20 mg/kg daily divided every 6 hr

PEDIATRIC

–PO: 30–50 mg/kg/day divided every 6 hr
–IV: 15–20 mg/kg daily divided every 4–6 hr

ADVERSE/SIDE EFFECTS

RAPID

–Anaphylaxis

GRADUAL

- Intestinal cramping and abdominal pain
- NVD
- Thrombophlebitis following IV infusion
- Stomatitis
- Overgrowth of nonsusceptible bacteria or fungi
- Urticaria, skin rash (rare)
- Hepatotoxicity
- Vaginitis
- Hearing loss

CONTRAINDICATIONS

- Hypersensitivity

SPECIAL PRECAUTIONS

- Pregnant or lactating patients
- Liver disease

OTHER SPECIAL INFORMATION

- To minimize GI distress, administer with 8 oz of water 1 hr before or 2 hr after meals.
- Intestinal cramping and abdominal pain usually subsides with continued dosing.
- Administer IV dose over 20–60 min; dilute each 250 mg in 100 ml of D_5W or NS.
- Reconstitute with sterile water without preservatives to prevent precipitation.

ANTIDOTE

SEVERE REACTIONS

- D/C drug immediately and initiate appropriate treatment for symptoms.
- Treat anaphylaxis with EPINEPHRINE, AMINOPHYLLINE, OXYGEN, IV corticosteroids.

OTHER REACTIONS

- Notify physician of any side effects and initiate appropriate actions.

ESMOLOL HCL Brevibloc

CLASS
–Beta-adrenergic blocker

USES
–Supraventricular tachycardia
–Noncompensatory tachycardia

ACTION
–Blocks beta-1 receptor site stimulation, reducing heart rate, contractility, AV conduction and O_2 consumption in myocardium
–Lowers blood pressure

USUAL DOSAGE/ROUTE
ADULT
–IV: 50–250 mcg/kg/min, not to exceed 200 mcg/kg/min
PEDIATRIC
–Safe use in children younger than age 18 not established

ADVERSE/SIDE EFFECTS
RAPID
–Induration (redness and elevated skin)
–Site inflammation
–Hypotension
–Bronchospasm
GRADUAL
–N & V
–Edema
–Pallor
–Confusion
–Urinary retention

CONTRAINDICATIONS
–Hypersensitivity
–Second- or third-degree heart block

–Cardiogenic shock
–Bradycardia
–Not for chronic use

SPECIAL PRECAUTIONS

–Pregnant or lactating patients
–Thyrotoxicosis (thyroid crisis)
–Hyperglycemia
–Hypotension

OTHER SPECIAL INFORMATION

–Monitor vital signs; notify physician if systolic BP greater than 100 or diastolic BP less than 60.
–Do not give if apical pulse is less than 60.
–Monitor respirations for changes in pattern or bronchospasm.

ANTIDOTE

SEVERE REACTIONS

–D/C drug immediately and initiate appropriate treatment for symptoms.

OTHER REACTIONS

–Notify physician of any side effects and initiate appropriate actions.

FAMOTIDINE Pepcid

CLASS
–Histamine H_2-receptor antagonist

USES
–Treatment of gastric ulcers
–Active duodenal ulcers
–Gastric hypersecretion such as Zollinger–Ellison syndrome

ACTION
–Inhibits action of histamine at H_2-receptor sites in gastric parietal cells to inhibit gastric acid secretion

USUAL DOSAGE/ROUTE

ADULT
–*Ulcers:* PO: 40 mg at bedtime or 20 mg 2 times/day for 2–8 weeks, then 20 mg at bedtime
–*Hypersecretion:* PO: 20 mg every 6 hr up to a maximum dose of 640 mg/day
–*Ulcers:* IV: 20 mg every 12 hr over at least 2 min diluted push or 15–30-min infusion
–*Hypersecretion:* IV: 20 mg every 6 hr over at least 2 min diluted push or 15–30 min infusion

PEDIATRIC
–Safe use in children not established

ADVERSE/SIDE EFFECTS

RAPID
–Rash
–Dizziness
–Headache
–Bronchospasm

GRADUAL
–Constipation
–Palpitations
–Muscle pain

–Reduced sexual desire
–Abnormal liver enzymes

CONTRAINDICATIONS
–Hypersensitivity

SPECIAL PRECAUTIONS
–Pregnant or lactating patients
–Renal impairment
–Liver impairment
–Elderly

OTHER SPECIAL INFORMATION
–Monitor for decreased platelet count frequently while using this drug.
–Monitor for thrombocytopenia, bruising, fatigue, bleeding.
–Peak = 1–3 hr, half-life = 2.5–3.5 hr.
–Dilute IV push drug with 5–10 ml of water for injection.

ANTIDOTE

SEVERE REACTIONS
–D/C drug immediately and initiate appropriate treatment for symptoms.

OTHER REACTIONS
–Notify physician of any side effects and initiate appropriate actions.

FAT EMULSION INFUSION (intravenous) Intralipid, Lyposyn II, Lyposyn III, Nutrilipid, Soyacal, Travamulsion (all solutions either 10% or 20%)

CLASS
–Fat emulsion (nonprotein calorie source)

USES

- Provides additional calories and essential fatty acids to clients receiving hyperalimentation infusions (total parenteral nutrition)
- Preventions for essential fatty acid deficiency

ACTION

- Supplies emulsified essential fatty acids (fat, phospholipid, and glycerol) for metabolism and use as a source of energy
- Increases heat production and oxygen consumption, and decreases respiratory quotient

USUAL DOSAGE/ROUTE

ADULT

- TPN Supplement: 500 ml of 10% or 250 ml of 20% IV daily over 4–6 hr using an infusion pump. Increase dose gradually each day, not exceeding 60% of the client's total caloric intake, or 2.5 gm/kg body weight.
- *Fatty acid deficiency:* Supply 8–10% of the total caloric intake with an IV infusion each 24 hr.

PEDIATRIC

- TPN Supplement: Infuse up to 1 gm/kg body weight IV daily over 4–6 hr using an infusion pump. Increase dose gradually each day, not exceeding 60% of total caloric intake or 4 gm/kg/day. Do not exceed a rate of 100 ml/hr (10%) or 50 ml/m (20%).

ADVERSE/SIDE EFFECTS

RAPID

- Anaphylaxis
- Chest pain
- Back pain
- Cyanosis
- Dizziness
- Dyspnea
- Flushing
- N & V

GRADUAL
- Elevated temperature
- Headache
- Hypercoagulability
- Hyperlipemia
- Pressure over eyes
- Sepsis
- Sleepiness
- Sweating
- Thrombophlebitis
- Focal seizures
- Leukocytosis
- Splenomegaly
- Shock
- Many others

CONTRAINDICATIONS
- Hypersensitivity
- Hyperlipemia
- Lipoid nephrosis
- Acute pancreatitis
- Severe egg allergies

SPECIAL PRECAUTIONS
- Pregnancy
- Pulmonary disease
- Anemia
- Patients with blood coagulation disorders
- Jaundiced or premature infants
- Infants and neonates
- When there is any danger of fat embolism

OTHER SPECIAL INFORMATION
- This drug may be administered IV by central or peripheral venous infusion since the drug is isotonic.
- Do not mix with any other IV solution or medication (except HEPARIN) and administer using a separate IV port.
- HEPARIN SODIUM 1–2 units/ml may be added to the IV emulsion to activate lipoprotein lipase.
- Do not use a filter with administration of this drug.

–This drug may be stored in the refrigerator at 77°–86°F (25°–30°C).
–Monitor liver function, Hgb, PT, PTT, plasma lipids, platelet count frequently during use.

ANTIDOTE

SEVERE REACTIONS
–D/C drug immediately and initiate appropriate treatment for symptoms.
–Initiate ALS protocols and resuscitate as necessary.

OTHER REACTIONS
–Notify physician of any side effects and initiate appropriate actions.
–Treat symptomatically.

FENTANYL CITRATE WITH DROPERIDOL
Innovar, Sublimaze

CLASS
–Preanesthetic, general anesthetic, narcotic analgesic

USES
–To produce analgesia and tranquilization for surgical and diagnostic procedures
–A preoperative medication for the induction of anesthesia and as an adjunct in the maintenance of general anesthesia
–Closed reduction of orthopedic injuries

ACTION
–Combines FENTANYL (a narcotic analgesic) and DROPERIDOL (a tranquilizer) to produce reduced motor activity, anesthesia; *Note:* complete loss of consciousness does not usually occur with use of this drug alone; incidence of early postoperative pain and emesis may be reduced.

USUAL DOSAGE/ROUTE

ADULT

–*Preoperative medication* IM: 0.5–2.0 ml IM 45–60 min before surgery
–*Adjunct to general anesthesia* IV: 1 ml/20–25 lb IV slowly over 3–4 min
–*Use without general anesthesia for diagnostic procedures* IM: 0.5–2.0 ml 45–60 min before procedure
–*Adjunct to regional anesthesia* IM or slow IV: 1–2 ml

PEDIATRIC

–*Preoperative medication* IM: 0.25 ml/20 lb 45–60 min before surgery with or without ATROPINE
–*Adjunct to general anesthesia* IV: 0.5 ml/20 lb

ADVERSE/SIDE EFFECTS

RAPID

–Respiratory depression, arrest
–Laryngospasm
–Bronchospasm
–Fine tremors
–Drowsiness
–Tachycardia
–Hypotension
–Muscle rigidity

GRADUAL

–Depression
–N & V
–Facial sweating & diaphoresis

CONTRAINDICATIONS

–Hypersensitivity to any combination of the drug
–Children under 2 years
–Myasthenia gravis

SPECIAL PRECAUTIONS

–Elderly
–Children
–Increased intracranial pressure

–Cardiovascular disease (brady dysrhythmias)
–Renal disease
–Liver disease
–Parkinson's disease
–COPD
–Pregnant or lactating patients

OTHER SPECIAL INFORMATION
–Because respiratory depression of this drug lasts longer than many drugs, postoperative pain narcotic dosages should be reduced to ¼–⅓ of usual dosages for 8–12 hr.
–Observe patients carefully for hypoventilation.
–Keep resuscitative equipment near and encourage recovering patient to take breaths on his or her own.

ANTIDOTE
SEVERE REACTIONS
–D/C drug immediately and initiate appropriate treatment for symptoms.
–Treat extrapyramidal reactions with anticholinergics such as DIPHENHYDRAMINE.
–Treat cardiac/respiratory arrest with advanced life support procedures as appropriate.
OTHER REACTIONS
–Notify physician of any side effects and initiate appropriate actions.

FLUORESCEIN SODIUM Fluor-I-Strip and others

CLASS
–Diagnostic ophthalmic fluorescent dye

USES
–Diagnostic in fitting hard contact lenses, lacrimal patency, corneal abrasions, foreign bodies, etc.
–Retinal angiography

ACTION

–Produces intense green fluorescent color in alkaline solution (pH 5 or greater) or bright yellow if viewed with cobalt blue illumination
–Assumes green color in presence of corneal epithelium break
–After IV administration, skin becomes yellow

USUAL DOSAGE/ROUTE

ADULT AND PEDIATRIC

–Topical: 1 drop of a 2% solution followed by irrigation with sterile water; have patient blink several times

ADULT (retinal angiography)

–IV: In retinal angiography, 5 ml of a 10% solution (500 mg) injected rapidly into antecubital vein by physician

PEDIATRIC

–IV: 0.077 ml of a 10% solution (7.7 mcg/kg) injected rapidly into antecubital vein by physician

ADVERSE/SIDE EFFECTS

RAPID

–Stinging and burning of the eye with topical use
–Yellowish skin discoloration persisting 6–12 hr after IV injection
–Anaphylaxis
–Convulsions
–Shock
–Cardiac arrest
–Acute pulmonary edema
–Dyspnea
–Headache persisting for 24–36 hr after IV use
–N & V
–Extravasation and thrombophlebitis at injection site
–Hypersensitivity reaction

GRADUAL

–None known

CONTRAINDICATIONS

–Hypersensitivity

SPECIAL PRECAUTIONS

–Bronchial asthma
–Pregnant or lactating patients

OTHER SPECIAL INFORMATION

–To avoid burning and stinging of eyes, instill topical anesthetic before FLUORESCEIN SODIUM.
–Perform a test dose (IV) before angiography is begun.
–A water-soluble dye is excreted in urine after IV injection.
–Use aseptic technique.
–Have anaphylaxis equipment and medications handy before IV administration.
–With topical instillation, corneal defects will appear green under normal light or bright yellow under cobalt blue illumination; foreign bodies are surrounded by a green ring and lesions of the conjunctiva are delineated in orange–yellow.

ANTIDOTE

SEVERE REACTIONS

–D/C drug immediately and initiate appropriate treatment for symptoms.
–Treat anaphylaxis with EPINEPHRINE, OXYGEN, and an antihistamine.

OTHER REACTIONS

–Notify physician of any side effects and initiate appropriate actions.

FUROSEMIDE Lasix, Myrosemide, Novosemide, Uritol

CLASS

–Loop diuretic (sulfonamide derivative)

USES

–Treatment of edema associated with CHF, cirrhosis of the liver, and renal hypertension

–Adjunct therapy in acute pulmonary edema
–Treatment for hypertension

ACTION

–Inhibits reabsorption of sodium and chloride in proximal and distal tubules and Henle's loop

USUAL DOSAGE/ROUTE

ADULT

–PO: 40–80 mg as a single dose; may be increased by 40 mg every 6–8 hr until desired diuresis obtained up to 600 mg/day
–IM, IV: 20–40 mg as a single dose increased by 20 mg every 2 hr until desired response

PEDIATRIC

–PO: 2 mg/kg body weight as a single dose; dosage may increase 1–2 mg/kg every 6–8 hr, but not to exceed 6 mg/kg/24 hr
–IM, IV: 1 mg/kg, not to exceed 6 mg/kg as a single dose, may increase by 1–2 mg/kg every 6–8 hr up to 6 mg/kg

ADVERSE/SIDE EFFECTS

RAPID

–Urinary frequency
–Rash, pruritis
–Hyperglycemia
–Circulatory collapse

GRADUAL

–Blurred vision
–Postural hypotension
–N & V
–Weakness
–Dizziness
–Muscle cramps
–Thirst
–Hypokalemia
–Hyponatremia
–Hypochloremia
–Thrombocytopenia

CONTRAINDICATIONS
–Hypersensitivity to sulfonamides
–Anuria
–Pregnancy and lactation
–Hypovolemia
–Persons with hepatic coma
–Infants
–In cases of excessive potassium loss & depletion of other electrolytes

SPECIAL PRECAUTIONS
–Diabetes mellitus
–Dehydration
–Ascites
–Severe renal disease

OTHER SPECIAL INFORMATION
–Monitor urinary output and blood pressure frequently with use.
–Administer IV at a rate of 10 mg/min.
–Monitor for signs and symptoms of hypokalemia (fatigue, weakness, anorexia, dehydration, abdominal distention, absent or decreased peristalsis, oliguria).
–PO: Onset = 1 hr; peak = 1–2 hr; duration = 6–8 hr.
–IM, IV: Onset = 5 min; peak = 30 min; duration = 2 hr.

ANTIDOTE

SEVERE REACTIONS
–D/C drug immediately and initiate appropriate treatment for symptoms
–Lavage stomach if taken orally
–Treat hyperglycemic reactions with an IV of dextrose and saline and insulin SQ and IV.

OTHER REACTIONS
–Notify physician of any side effects and initiate appropriate actions.

GENTAMYCIN SULFATE Garamycin and others

CLASS
–Aminoglycoside antibiotic

USES
–Severe local and systemic infections caused by pseudomonas aeruginosa, Escherichia coli, proteus, klebsiella, serratia, enterobacteriaceae staphylococcus

ACTION
–Inhibits protein synthesis of the bacterial cells in susceptible organisms

USUAL DOSAGE/ROUTE
ADULT (with normal renal function)
–IM, IV: 3 mg/kg/day in divided doses every 8 hr; may receive up to 5 mg/kg/day in 3–4 divided doses

PEDIATRIC (with normal renal function)
–IM, IV: 2–2.5 mg/kg every 8 hr
–IM, IV (infants over 1 week): 2.5 mg/kg every 8 hr
–IV (infants under 1 week): 2.5 mg/kg every 12 hr

ADVERSE/SIDE EFFECTS
RAPID
–Convulsions
–N & V
–Rash, urticaria

GRADUAL
–Nephrotoxicity
–Ototoxicity
–Blood dyscrasias
–Hematuria
–Oliguria
–Neuromuscular blockade with respiratory failure

–Thrombocytopenia
–Anorexia

CONTRAINDICATIONS
–Hypersensitivity
–Severe renal disease

SPECIAL PRECAUTIONS
–Neonates
–Elderly
–Mild renal disease
–Hearing deficits
–Myasthenia gravis
–Pregnant or lactating patients

OTHER SPECIAL INFORMATION
–Patient with impaired renal function: initial dose is same for those with normal function; subsequent doses are to be determined by blood level monitoring.
–Mix IV dose with 50–200 ml D_5W or NS and infuse over 30 minutes.
–Monitor and evaluate renal function before and during therapy.
–Evaluate patient's hearing before and during therapy.
–Activity against pseudomonas increases when used concurrently with CARBENICILLIN.
–Do not dose according to total body weight in patients who exceed ideal body weight by 100%; use ideal weight plus 40% of fat weight.
–Monitor and evaluate serum levels frequently in elderly patients and patients with renal or hepatic dysfunction.

ANTIDOTE

SEVERE REACTIONS
–D/C drug immediately and initiate appropriate treatment for symptoms.
–Treat anaphylaxis with dialysis and appropriate advanced life support procedures

OTHER REACTIONS

–Notify physician of any side effects and initiate appropriate actions.

GLUCAGON, USP Glucagon

CLASS

–Insulin antagonist (hormone)

USES

–To increase glucose levels in hypoglycemia (insulin shock)
–To terminate insulin-induced shock in psychiatric patients
–Diagnostic aid in radiologic examination of stomach, duodenum, small bowel, and colon (relaxes esophagus)

ACTION

–Glucagon is a protein produced by the alpha cells of the pancreas that mobilizes glucose stored in the liver and simulates the manufacture of neoglucose from fats.
–Relaxes smooth muscles of the stomach, duodenum, small bowel, and colon

USUAL DOSAGE/ROUTE

ADULT

–SC, IM, IV: 0.5–1.0 mg and may repeat within 20 min × 2

PEDIATRIC

–SC, IM, IV: 0.5–1.0 mg and may repeat within 20 min × 2

ADVERSE/SIDE EFFECTS

RAPID

–Hypersensitivity reactions
–N & V

GRADUAL

–None known

CONTRAINDICATIONS

–Hypersensitivity
–Renal disease
–Liver disease
–Undernourished and/or emaciated patients
–Insulin-Dependent Diabetic Mellitus (IDDM) patients

SPECIAL PRECAUTIONS

–History of insulinoma (tumor of the islets of the pancreas)
–History of pheochromocytoma (adrenal gland tumor)

OTHER SPECIAL INFORMATION

–This drug precipitates when mixed with CHLORIDE solutions.
–This drug is effective in overcoming hypoglycemia only when the liver has a reserve of glycogen.
–Large doses of this drug may enhance the effect of oral anticoagulants.
–Give carbohydrates as soon as the patient awakens to prevent secondary hypoglycemic reactions.
–EPINEPHRINE intensifies and prolongs the hyperglycemic effect of this drug.
–If the patient does not respond to treatment in 5–20 minutes, proceed with administering IV dextrose.
–Onset = 5–20 min; peak = 30 min; duration = 1–2 hr.

ANTIDOTE

SEVERE REACTIONS

–D/C drug immediately and initiate appropriate treatment for symptoms.
–Treat hypoglycemia with 20% or 50% dextrose injection and follow up with IV dextrose solution while stabilizing blood glucose levels.

OTHER REACTIONS

–Notify physician of any side effects and initiate appropriate actions.

GLYBURIDE Micronase

CLASS
–Oral hypoglycemic (sulfonylurea)

USES
–Control of blood sugar levels in adult onset, non-insulin-dependent diabetes

ACTION
–Stimulates release of insulin from the beta cells of the pancreas; increases sensitivity of insulin at receptor sites; lowers blood sugar

USUAL DOSAGE/ROUTE
ADULT
–PO: 2.5–5.0 mg daily in one dose, at breakfast, not to exceed 10 mg per dose up to a maximum of 20 mg/day

PEDIATRIC
–Not for use in children

ADVERSE/SIDE EFFECTS
RAPID
–Hypoglycemia
–Rash

GRADUAL
–Tachycardia
–Weakness
–Headache
–Nausea/heartburn
–Hepatotoxicity
–Cholestatic jaundice
–Leukopenia
–Thrombocytopenia
–Aplastic anemia
–Dry mouth
–Urinary hesitancy

CONTRAINDICATIONS

–Hypersensitivity to sulfonylureas or thiazides
–Pregnant or lactating patients
–Insulin-dependent diabetes
–Severe renal impairment
–Hepatic impairment
–Thyroid disease
–Burns
–Acidosis
–Severe infection
–Severe trauma

SPECIAL PRECAUTIONS

–Elderly
–Malnourished patients
–Liver insufficiency
–Renal insufficiency
–Thyroid impairment
–Adrenal impairment
–Pituitary impairment

OTHER SPECIAL INFORMATION

–Infection or dietary changes may alter dosage needed.
–Effects decrease with DIAZOXIDE.
–Decreases digoxin levels.
–Hypoglycemic effects increase with CIMETIDINE, INSULIN, MAO inhibitors, oral anticoagulants, methyldopa, NSAID, salicylates, PROBENECID, and CHLORAMPHENICOL.
–Effect decreases with calcium channel blockers, corticosteroids, oral contraceptives, thiazide diuretics, thyroid preparations, estrogens, phenothiazides, PHENYTOIN, PHENOBARBITAL, RIFAMPIN, ISONIAZIDE, sympathomimetics.
–Do not use with alcohol.
–Tablets may be crushed and taken with fluids.
–Serum blood sugar levels must be monitored when taking this drug.

ANTIDOTE

SEVERE REACTIONS

–D/C drug immediately and initiate appropriate treatment for symptoms.

–Overdose: 10–50% glucose sol or 1 mg GLUCAGON IV.

OTHER REACTIONS

–Notify physician of side effects; initiate appropriate actions.

GUANFACINE HCL   Tenex

CLASS

–Antihypertensive (alpha-2 adrenergic receptor agonist)

USES

–Used with thiazide diuretics to manage hypertension

ACTION

–Lowers blood pressure by stimulating alpha-adrenergic receptors which decreases sympathetic outflow, decreases peripheral vascular resistance and slightly lowers heart rate

USUAL DOSAGE/ROUTE

ADULT

–PO: 0.5–1.0 mg/day at bedtime, may increase dosage at 3–4-week intervals up to 3 mg/day

PEDIATRIC

–Not for use in children

ADVERSE/SIDE EFFECTS

RAPID

–Hypotension

–NVD

–Dyspnea

–Faintness
–Bradycardia

GRADUAL

–Drowsiness
–Weakness
–Orthostatic hypotension
–Palpitations
–Chest pain
–Dry mouth
–Constipation
–Leg cramps
–Impotence
–Headache
–Insomnia
–Depression

CONTRAINDICATIONS

–Hypersensitivity
–Severe depression
–Suicidal tendencies

SPECIAL PRECAUTIONS

–Severe coronary disease
–Recent myocardial infarction
–Pregnant or lactating patients
–Renal disease
–Liver disease
–CVA
–Children < 12 years
–History of mental depression

OTHER SPECIAL INFORMATION

–Increases hypotension if used with other antihypertensive agents
–Increases CNS depression if used with CNS depressants such as alcohol, antihistamines, and sedatives/hypnotics
–Decreases hypotensive effects if used with tricyclic antihypertensives, phenothiazines, EPHIDRINE, PHENYLPROPANOLAMINE, oral contraceptives, HALOPERIDOL, amphetamines

–Do not discontinue drug abruptly, will cause withdrawal symptoms

ANTIDOTE

SEVERE REACTIONS

–D/C drug immediately and initiate appropriate treatment for symptoms.

–Treat respiratory/cardiac side effects with ISOPROTERENOL.

OTHER REACTIONS

–Notify physician of any side effects and initiate appropriate actions.

HALOPERIDOL USP, HALOPERIDOL DECANOATE Haldol, Peridol

CLASS
–Antipsychotic, tranquilizer

USES
–Treatment of psychotic and schizophrenic disorders, Gilles de la Tourette's syndrome, management of behavioral problems in mental deficiency, and as an alternative medication for persons hypersensitive to phenothiazines
–Short-term treatment of hyperactive children showing excessive motor activity

ACTION
–Depresses cerebral cortex, hypothalamus, limbic system to control activity and aggression; blocks neurotransmission produced by dopamine at synapse; action similar to phenothiazine tranquilizers in treatment of psychosis

USUAL DOSAGE/ROUTE
ADULT
–PO: 0.5–5.0 mg 2–3 times/day up to a maximum dose of 100 mg/day
–IM: 2–5 mg every 1–8 hr depending on severity of condition
–*Chronic schizophrenia:* IM: 10–15 times the PO dose every 4th week (DECANOATE)

PEDIATRIC (3–12 yr)
–PO, IM: 0–.05–0.15 mg/kg/day

ADVERSE/SIDE EFFECTS
RAPID
–Laryngospasm
–Respiratory depression
–Dyspnea
–Seizures
–Rash

–Dry mouth
–Cardiac arrest
–Tachycardia

GRADUAL

–Extrapyramidal reactions: Parkinson-like symptoms, motor restlessness, dystonia
–Euphoria
–Hyperreflexia
–Insomnia
–Transient leukopenia and leukocytosis
–Impaired liver function
–Anorexia
–Constipation
–NVD
–Orthostatic hypotension
–Tardive dyskinesia

CONTRAINDICATIONS

–Hypersensitivity
–Severe CNS depression
–Comatose states
–Blood dyscrasias
–Children younger than 3 yr
–Parkinson's disease
–Bone marrow depression
–Epilepsy
–Urinary retention

SPECIAL PRECAUTIONS

–Pregnant or lactating patients
–Seizure disorders
–Hypertension
–Liver disease
–Cardiac disease

OTHER SPECIAL INFORMATION

–Drug decreases the effectiveness of anticoagulants and anticonvulsants.
–IM: Onset = 15–30 min; peak = 15–20 min; half-life = 21 hr.

–IM (DECANOATE): Peak = 4–11 days; half-life = 3 weeks.
–Drug can be used in treatment of intractable nausea from radiation or chemotherapy.
–Drug can be used in management of chronic pain.

ANTIDOTE

SEVERE REACTIONS

–D/C drug immediately and initiate appropriate treatment for symptoms.
–Treat extrapyramidal reactions with anticholinergics such as DIPHENHYDRAMINE or ATROPINE or anti-Parkinsonism agent.
–Treat cardiac arrest with ALS procedures as appropriate
–Induce emesis and give ACTIVATED CHARCOAL if orally ingested.

OTHER REACTIONS

–Notify physician of any side effects and initiate appropriate actions.

HEPARIN SODIUM Calciparine, Heparin, Hep Lock

CLASS

–Anticoagulant

USES

–Prophylaxis and treatment of venous thrombosis
–Treatment of pulmonary embolism, disseminated intravascular coagulation, coronary occlusion
–Prevention of cerebral thrombosis in stroke, clotting in arterial and heart surgery

ACTION

–Prolongs the clotting time of blood by preventing fibrin clot formation and inhibiting the conversion of prothrombin to thrombin

USUAL DOSAGE/ROUTE

ADULT (prophylaxis for thromboembolism)

–SC: 5,000 U every 8–12 hr.

ADULT (deep vein thrombosis and MI)

–IV push: 5,000–7,000 U initially then titrate to PTT level every 4 hr.

–IV infusion: 5,000–7,000 U bolus then 1,000 U/hr titrated to PTT level

ADULT (pulmonary embolism)

–IV push: 7,500–10,000 U bolus then titrate to PTT level every 4 hr

–IV infusion: 7,500–10,000 U bolus, then 1,000 U/hr titrated to PTT level

ADULT (open heart surgery)

–IV infusion: 150–300 U/kg

–Heparin lock—IV push: 5–100 U/0.5–1 ml after each medication or every 8–12 hr

PEDIATRIC (all conditions)

–IV infusion: 5O U/kg then maintain on 100 U/kg every 4 hr or 20,000 U/M^2/day

–Heparin lock—IV push: 5–100 U/0.5–1 ml after each medication or every 8–12 hr

ADVERSE/SIDE EFFECTS

RAPID

–Hematoma
–Pain or irritation at injection site
–Rash, urticaria, pruritus

GRADUAL

–Hemorrhage
–GI or urinary tract bleeding
–Bleeding gums
–Epistaxis
–Diarrhea
–Hepatitis
–Alopecia
–Fever, chills
–Thrombocytopenia

CONTRAINDICATIONS
–In persons with hypersensitivity to HEPARIN
–Hemophilia
–Leukemia
Peptic ulcer disease
–Hepatic disease
–Renal disease

SPECIAL PRECAUTIONS
–Alcoholism
–Elderly
–Pregnancy

OTHER SPECIAL INFORMATION
–This drug is not effective by oral administration.
–With deep subcutaneous injections, rotate injection sites to lessen tissue damage; do not give IM.
–SC onset = 20–60 min; duration = 8–12 hr; IV onset = 5–10 min; duration = 2–6 hr.
–Pain at injection sites may be lessened by cold compresses or ice cubes.
–Monitor for unexpected bleeding; advise patients to avoid use of sharp instruments (hand razors) or strenuous activities that may incur tissue damage (contact sports).
–Monitor lab studies frequently (PTT) for adequate clotting time of approximately 1½–2 times the control.
–Do not massage area or aspirate when giving SC injection (minimizes tissue injury and bleeding).
–Chronic long-term use may lead to bone demineralization.

ANTIDOTE

SEVERE REACTIONS
–D/C drug immediately and initiate appropriate treatment for symptoms.
–Treat bleeding with the antidote PROTAMINE SULFATE.

OTHER REACTIONS
–Notify physician of any side effects and initiate appropriate actions.

HETASTARCH HES, Hespan, Hydroxyethyl Starch

CLASS
–Plasma volume expander (synthetic polymer)

USES
–Adjunct in the early management of shock or impending shock due to burns, bleeding, surgery, or sepsis
–Fluid replacement and plasma volume expansion in trauma
–Leukapheresis

ACTION
–A synthetic molecule that acts like a colloidal osmotic agent similar to human albumin to expand plasma volume by colloidal osmotic pressure

USUAL DOSAGE/ROUTE

ADULT
–IV infusion: 500–1000 ml (30–60 gm of a 6% solution), not to exceed 1500 ml/day, or 20 ml/kg/hr
–*Leukapheresis:* IV infusion: 250–700 ml infused at 1:8 ratio with whole blood and may repeat every 2 weeks up to 10 treatments

PEDIATRIC
–Safe use in children not established

ADVERSE/SIDE EFFECTS

RAPID
–Anaphylaxis
–Decreased hematocrit
–Bronchospasm
–PE
–N & V
–Rash
–Urticaria
–Pruritis

–Chills/fever
–Flushing
–Wheezing
–Dyspnea

GRADUAL
–Increased coagulation/bleeding times
–Headache
–Increased urine output
–Circulatory overload
–Dehydration

CONTRAINDICATIONS
–Hypersensitivity
–Severe bleeding disorders
–CHF, severe CHF/PE
–Renal failure with anuria or oliguria

SPECIAL PRECAUTIONS
–Pregnant or lactating patients
–Thrombocytopenia
–Liver disease
–Elderly
–Children

OTHER SPECIAL INFORMATION
–Assess patient for signs of vascular overload (elevated CVP, rales/crackles, dyspnea, hypertension, jugular vein distention).
–Assess patient for increased bleeding caused by interference with platelet function and clotting factors.
–Drug may cause an increase in PT, PTT, ESR, and clotting times.
–Do not administer if the solution is cloudy or contains precipitate.
–Crossmatching is not required because there is no danger of serum hepatitis or AIDS.
–Administer undiluted by IV infusion.

ANTIDOTE

SEVERE REACTIONS

–D/C drug immediately and initiate appropriate treatment for symptoms.

OTHER REACTIONS

–Notify physician of any side effects and initiate appropriate actions.

HYDRALAZINE HCL Alazine, Apresoline, Dralzine, Rolzine

CLASS

–Antihypertensive (vasodilator)

USES

–Moderate-to-severe hypertension
–Increased cardiac output (direct inotropic effect)
–Increased renal blood flow
–CHF unresponsive to cardiac glycosides and diuretics (decreases afterload)

ACTION

–Acts directly on peripheral arteriolar smooth muscle causing vasodilation

USUAL DOSAGE/ROUTE

ADULT

–PO: Initial 10–25 mg daily; daily dose may increase by 10–25 mg until desired effect achieved; maximal daily dose is 400 mg in 4 divided doses
–IM, IV: 10–20 mg increased to 40 mg repeated as necessary every 4–6 hr

PEDIATRIC

–PO: 0.75 mg/kg/day in 4 divided doses; may be increased up to 7.5 mg/kg/day over a two-week period
–IM, IV: 1.7–3.5 mg/kg/day in 4–6 divided doses

ADVERSE/SIDE EFFECTS

RAPID

–Hypotension
–Headache
–Tachycardia
–Palpitations
–Dizziness
–Faintness
–Malaise
–Angina
–NVD
–Shock

GRADUAL

–Lupus-like symptoms.
–Anorexia
–Leukopenia
–Agranulocytosis
–Impotence
–Urinary retention
–Sodium & water retention

CONTRAINDICATIONS

–Hypersensitivity
–Coronary artery disease
–Mitral valvular rheumatic heart disease

SPECIAL PRECAUTIONS

–Pregnant or lactating patients
–Advanced renal disease
–CVA patients

OTHER SPECIAL INFORMATION

–Lower dosages are often given in combination with other drugs due to increased side effects of this drug.
–Do not mix this drug with any other drug in the syringe or in a solution.
–Administer PO tablets with meals to lessen gastric irritability.
–Drug-induced lupus-like syndrome occurs in 10–20% of patients, especially those receiving greater than 200 mg/

day; this syndrome occurs almost exclusively in Caucasians who are slow acetylators; syndrome is completely reversible.

ANTIDOTE

SEVERE REACTIONS

–D/C drug immediately and initiate appropriate treatment for symptoms.

–Lavage the patient if this drug is taken orally, then administer ACTIVATED CHARCOAL.

–Treat hypotension with vasopressors such as DOPAMINE.

–Treat shock with volume expanders and digitalization.

OTHER REACTIONS

–Notify physician of any side effects and initiate appropriate actions.

HYDROCHLOROTHIAZIDE, USP

Chlorzide, Esidrix, Hydrodiuril, Hydrozide, Oretic, and others

CLASS

–Thiazide diuretic, antihypertensive (sulfonamide derivative)

USES

–Treatment of hypertension, alone or in combination with other antihypertensive agents

–Treatment of fluid retention, congestive heart failure, renal edema, premenstrual tension, glomerulonephritis

ACTION

–Affects the renal tubular mechanisms of electrolyte reabsorption

–Increases excretion of sodium and chloride and potassium at the distal tubule of the kidneys

–Antihypertensive effect mechanism unknown

USUAL DOSAGE/ROUTE

ADULT

–PO: 25–100 mg/day in 1–2 divided doses not exceeding 200 mg/day

PEDIATRIC

–(more than 6 mos) PO: 2.2 mg/kg/day in 2 divided doses
–(less than 6 mos) PO: up to 3.3 mg/kg/day in 2 divided doses

ADVERSE/SIDE EFFECTS

RAPID

–Rashes
–Weakness
–Restlessness
–Dizziness
–Vertigo

GRADUAL

–NVD
–Leukopenia
–Agranulocytosis
–Orthostatic hypotension
–Hypotension
–Hyperglycemia
–Hypokalemia
–Hyponatremia
–Hypercalcemia
–Hypovolemia
–Photosensitivity
–Muscle spasm
–Hyperuricemia and/or gout
–Pancreatitis

CONTRAINDICATIONS

–Hypersensitivity to this or other sulfonamide drugs
–Anuria
–Lactation

SPECIAL PRECAUTIONS
–Pregnant or lactating patients
–Renal disease
–Liver disease

OTHER SPECIAL INFORMATION
–Monitor intake and output.
–Record daily weight.
–Monitor uric acid, BUN, sodium, and potassium blood levels.
–Monitor blood pressure.
–Dosages in excess of 100 mg/day for hypertension exceed maximal effect and only lead to side effects.

ANTIDOTE
SEVERE REACTIONS
–D/C drug immediately and initiate appropriate treatment for symptoms
OTHER REACTIONS
–Notify physician of any side effects and initiate appropriate actions.

HYDROCORTISONE, HYDROCORTISONE ACETATE, HYDROCORTISONE SODIUM PHOSPHATE, HYDROCORTISONE SODIUM SUCCINATE Cortef, Hydrocortone, Solu Cortef, and others

CLASS
–Short-acting corticosteroid (glucocorticoid)

USES
–Severe inflammation
–Adrenal insufficiency
–Shock
–Ulcerative colitis

ACTION

–Concerned primarily with glucose metabolism; suppresses the normal immune response and inflammation

USUAL DOSAGE/ROUTE

ADULTS

–*Replacement:* PO: 10–25 mg daily
–*Anti-inflammatory:* PO: 40–80 mg daily
–IV: 100–250 mg slowly over 2 hr (SUCCINATE) or 15–240 mg every 12 hr (PHOSPHATE)
–IM: 50–100 mg as needed

PEDIATRIC

–IM, IV: 0.16–1.0 mg/kg 2–3 times/day (SUCCINATE)

ADVERSE/SIDE EFFECTS

RAPID

–Circulatory collapse
–Blurred vision
–Tachycardia
–Hypertension
–Sweating
–Flushing

GRADUAL

–Mood swings
–Depression
–Insomnia
–Poor wound healing
–Ecchymosis, petechiae
–Cataracts, glaucoma
–NVD
–Peptic ulcer
–GI irritation
–Thrombophlebitis
–Iatrogenic hyperadrenocorticoidism
–Embolism
–Thrombocytopenia
–Pancreatitis

CONTRAINDICATIONS
–Hypersensitivity
–Peptic ulcer
–Psychosis
–Idiopathic thrombocytopenia
–Acute glomerulonephritis
–Cushing's syndrome
–Respiratory disease
–Systemic fungal infections
–Hypertension
–CHF

SPECIAL PRECAUTIONS
–Pregnant or lactating patients
–Diabetes mellitus
–Glaucoma
–Osteoporosis
–Seizure disorders
–Myasthenia gravis

OTHER SPECIAL INFORMATION
–Gradually reduce drug dosage.
–Titrate to lowest effective dose.
–Discard reconstituted solutions after 48 hours.
–Monitor weight, BP, sleep patterns, serum electrolytes.
–Teach patient signs of early adrenal insufficiency (nausea, dyspnea, weakness, joint pain).
–Give IM deep into gluteal muscle.
–Give PO with food.
–Warn patients on long-term therapy about cushingoid symptoms.

ANTIDOTE

SEVERE REACTIONS
–D/C drug immediately and initiate appropriate treatment for symptoms.

OTHER REACTIONS
–Notify physician of any side effects and initiate appropriate actions.

HYDROMORPHONE HCL Dihydromorphinone, Dilaudid, Dilaudid-HP

CLASS
–Narcotic analgesic, antitussive

USES
–For relief of moderate-to-severe pain
–Antitussive in lower doses

ACTION
–Acts on sensory cortex to produce analgesia
–Enhances parasympathetic activity

USUAL DOSAGE/ROUTE

ADULT
–PO: 1–6 mg every 4–6 hr PRN
–IM, IV: 2–4 mg every 4–6 hr PRN
–SC: 2–4mg every 4–6 hr PRN
–Rectally: 3 mg every 4–8 hr PRN
–*Antitussive*: PO: 1 mg every 3–4 hr

PEDIATRIC (6–12 yr)
–*Antitussive*:PO: 0.5 mg every 3–4 hours

ADVERSE/SIDE EFFECTS

RAPID
–Hypotension
–N & V
–Sedation
–Respiratory depression
–Confusion
–Bradycardia

GRADUAL
–Physical and psychological dependence
–Constipation

CONTRAINDICATIONS
–Hypersensitivity
–Seizures
–Shock
–Migraine headaches

SPECIAL PRECAUTIONS
–Pregnant or lactating patients
–Head trauma
–Increased ICP
–Renal disease
–Liver disease
–Pulmonary disease
–Adrenal insufficiency
–Hypothyroidism
–Alcoholism
–Prostatic hypertrophy

OTHER SPECIAL INFORMATION
–Give IV dose over 3–5 minutes.
–6 times as potent (mg/mg SC dosing) as MORPHINE SULFATE.
–All drug forms onset = 10–30 min; peak = 15–45 min; duration = 2–5 hr.

ANTIDOTE

SEVERE REACTIONS
–D/C drug immediately and initiate appropriate treatment for symptoms.
–Treat overdose with NALOXONE IV push and IV infusion until desired result.

OTHER REACTIONS
–Notify physician of any side effects and initiate appropriate actions.

HYDROXYZINE HCL, HYDROXYZINE PAMOATE **Anxanil, Atarax, Atozine, Durrax, E-Vista, Hy-Pam, Orgatrax, Quiess, Vistaril, and others**

CLASS
–Antianxiety agent (minor tranquilizer), antihistamine

USES
–Anxiety due to psychoneurosis and organic disorders
–Antiemetic postoperatively
–Potentiate narcotic analgesics
–Pruritis, allergies, asthma, chronic urticaria when related to emotional overlay

ACTION
–Depresses key regions of the subcortical area of CNS including limbic system and reticular formation

USUAL DOSAGE/ROUTE
ADULT
–PO, IM: 25–100 mg 3–4 times/day
PEDIATRIC
–PO: 50–100 mg daily in divided doses
–IM: 1.1 mg/kg 3–4 times/day

ADVERSE/SIDE EFFECTS
RAPID
–Hypotension
–Dry mouth
–Dizziness
–Drowsiness
–Blurred vision
–Tremors
GRADUAL
–Fatigue
–Depression

CONTRAINDICATIONS
–Hypersensitivity
–Early pregnancy

SPECIAL PRECAUTIONS
–Elderly
–Debilitated
–Liver disease
–Renal disease

OTHER SPECIAL INFORMATION
–PO: Onset = 15–30 min; half-life = 3 hr; duration = 4–6 hr.
–Drug potentiates MEPERIDINE HCL and other CNS depressants, barbiturates, and alcohol.
–Drug has true intrinsic pain-relieving properties.
–Initial drug therapy may cause drowsiness.
–Drug is closely related to the antihistamines.
–Administer IM by Z-track to decrease pain and lessen chance of necrosis.
–Drug is first choice for histamine-related urticaria.

ANTIDOTE

SEVERE REACTIONS
–D/C drug immediately and initiate appropriate treatment for symptoms.
–Gastric: Lavage if orally ingested.
–Treat hypotension with NOREPINEPHRINE IV.

OTHER REACTIONS
–Notify physician of any side effects and initiate appropriate actions.

HYPERALIMENTATION INFUSION (intravenous), (PROTEIN PRODUCTS, AMINO ACID PRODUCTS) Aminess, Aminosyn, Aminosyn-M, Aminosyn II, Aminosyn PF, Aminosyn RF, Branch Amin, FreAmine HBC, HepaAmine, Nephramise, Total Parenteral Nutrition, Trarasol, and many other names in a variety of concentrations

CLASS
–Protein (amino acid) product for intravenous infusion

USES
–Restoration and maintenance of positive nitrogen balance in severe illness when oral intake is not practical or normal GI absorption is impaired

ACTION
–Supplies both essential and nonessential amino acids (protein) and calories to promote protein production, prevent protein breakdown, promote wound healing, and buffer body fluids

USUAL DOSAGE/ROUTE

ADULT

–Average is 2 liters/24 hr IV providing 1–2 gm protein/kg of body weight; dosage depends on individual protein needs, physical condition, and body weight. Begin administration at a rate of 1 liter/24 hr and gradually increase by 1 liter/24 hr to desired amount (infuse at 1–2 ml/kg/hr using an infusion pump and microfilter).

PEDIATRIC

–Average is 100–500 milliliters/24 hr IV providing 2–3 gm protein/kg of body weight; dosage depends on individual protein needs, physical condition, and body weight. Infuse at a constant rate evenly distributed over a 24-hr period using an infusion pump and microfilter.

ADVERSE/SIDE EFFECTS

RAPID

–Anaphylaxis
–Convulsions
–Abdominal pains
–Metabolic acidosis/alkalosis
–Vomiting

GRADUAL

–Bone demineralization
–Changes in LOC
–Dehydration
–Edema and phlebitis at IV site
–Electrolyte imbalances
–Hypertension
–Glycosuria
–Hyperaminonemia
–Hyperglycemia
–Hyperpyrexia
–Pulmonary edema
–Septicemia
–Weakness
–Vasodilation

CONTRAINDICATIONS

–Hypersensitivity to any component
–Acidosis
–Anuria
–Azotemia
–Low RBCs, Hgb
–Severe liver disease

SPECIAL PRECAUTIONS

–Diabetes mellitus
–Kidney disease
–Children and infants

OTHER SPECIAL INFORMATION

–Use promptly after mixing by strict aseptic technique under Laminar flow hood (may refrigerate briefly if necessary).
–Use only if solution is clear.
–Use large vein to infuse, usually central administration by subclavian or superior vena cava.
–Peripheral veins may be used for administration when amino acid products are diluted with 2.5%, 5%, or 10% dextrose.
–Use strict aseptic technique with regular IV site care.
–Do not use the infusion IV port to draw blood, transfuse blood, or administer other medications (pseudoagglutination and thrombosis can occur).
–Baseline studies are required prior to administration and frequently during administration (CBC, platelet count, PT, BUN, SMA-6, SMA-12, magnesium, phosphorus, body weight and length, and head circumference in infants).
–Measure urine glucose and ketones every 8 hr during infusion.
–Discontinue infusion if BUN exceeds normal limits and is continuing to rise.
–Additional insulin coverage may be required during administration.
–RDA vitamins, trace metals, and electrolytes must be supplemented with administration of this fluid.
–This fluid is frequently used in conjunction with an IV fat emulsion as a nonprotein calorie source, administered using a separate container and a separate IV port.
–Discard any unused solution after 24 hr.
–Replace IV administration set every 24–48 hr.

ANTIDOTE

SEVERE REACTIONS

–D/C drug immediately and initiate appropriate treatment for symptoms.
–Initiate ALS protocols and resuscitate as necessary

OTHER REACTIONS

–Notify physician of any side effects and initiate appropriate actions.

–An alternative brand, adjustment of additives, or a reduced rate may be required to prevent reactions.
–Treat symptomatically.

IBUPROFEN Amersol, Motrin, Rufen

CLASS
–Nonsteroidal anti-inflammatory (antirheumatic)

USES
–For relief of chronic symptoms associated with rheumatoid arthritis, osteoarthritis, and gout
–Relief of menstrual cramps/aches
–Relief of acute self-limiting minor-to-moderate pain

ACTION
–Possesses nonsteroidal anti-inflammatory effect as well as antipyretic and analgesic properties
–True mode of action not known
–Anti-inflammatory action possibly secondary to inhibition of prostaglandin synthesis and/or release
–Antipyretic effect thought to be associated with action on the hypothalamus

USUAL DOSAGE/ROUTE

ADULT
–PO: 300–600 mg 3–4 times/day; use smallest dosage necessary to control symptoms; total daily dosage should not exceed 2400 mg

PEDIATRIC
–Not for use in children 14 years of age or younger

ADVERSE/SIDE EFFECTS

RAPID
–Drowsiness
–Dry mouth
–Dizziness
–Pruritus/rash
–Blurred vision
–Tachycardia
–Dysrhythmias

GRADUAL
- –GI upset
- –NVD
- –Headachc
- –Tinnitus
- –Edema
- –Decreased Hgb and Hct
- –Leukopenia
- –Peptic ulcer
- –Insomnia
- –Anxiety
- –Depression
- –Nephrotoxicity
- –Blood dyscrasias

CONTRAINDICATIONS
- –Hypersensitivity to nonsteroidal anti-inflammatory drugs
- –Active peptic ulcer disease
- –Cardiac compromise/dysfunction
- –Children
- –Hepatic or renal insufficiency

SPECIAL PRECAUTIONS
- –Pregnant or lactating patients
- –Bleeding disorders
- –GI disorders

OTHER SPECIAL INFORMATION
- –This drug may be displaced by HYDANTOIN, SULFONAMIDES, or SULFONYLUREAS leading to toxicity.
- –Because this drug inhibits platelet aggregation, do not recommend use of oral anticoagulants with continuous use of this drug.
- –This drug may be administered with food or milk if GI intolerance occurs; however, absorption rate is slower and drug plasma level is reduced.
- –Concurrent aspirin usage may decrease the serum level and anti-inflammatory effects.

ANTIDOTE

SEVERE REACTIONS

–D/C drug immediately and initiate appropriate treatment for symptoms.

OTHER REACTIONS

–Notify physician of any side effects and initiate appropriate actions.

INSULIN Lente: Iletin I, Iletin II; NPH: NPH Isophane; Regular: Regular Iletin

CLASS

–Antidiabetic agent

USES

–Control of type I and type II diabetes mellitus, with insulin modified by the addition of zinc chloride and globin
–Ketoacidosis
–Useful in patients sensitive to protamine
–Occasionally used during hyperalimentation

ACTION

–Decreases blood sugar
–Stimulates carbohydrate metabolism by facilitating transport of glucose into the cell

USUAL DOSAGE/ROUTE

ADULT AND PEDIATRIC

–SC, IV: Individualized according to blood and urine glucose levels, diet and exercise; given subcutaneously by injection in morning before breakfast (usual dose 7–26 U)
–Lente and NPH insulin not suitable for IV administration

ADVERSE/SIDE EFFECTS

RAPID

–Anaphylaxis
–Excessive doses cause hypoglycemia
–Tachycardia
–Hypersensitivity to Lente Insulin
–Palpitations

GRADUAL

–Headache
–Weakness
–Fatigue

CONTRAINDICATIONS

–Hypersensitivity
–Insulin shock

SPECIAL PRECAUTIONS

–Pregnant or lactating patients

OTHER SPECIAL INFORMATION

–Mix well before administration by rolling vial between hands because Lente Insulin is a suspension.
–Normal blood glucose levels are approx 80–110 mg/dl.
–Rotate sites of injections.
–Educate patient regarding prescribed diet, signs and symptoms of hypoglycemia and hyperglycemia, medication care and administration, importance of regular check-ups for blood glucose levels.
–Regular insulin may be given IV or SC; onset = ½–1 hr; peak = 2–4 hr; duration = 5–7 hr.
–Lente Insulin: SC: onset = 1–3 hr; peak = 6–12 hr; duration = 24–28 hr.
–NPH Insulin: SC: onset = 1–3 hr; peak = 6–12 hr; duration = 24–28 hr.

ANTIDOTE

SEVERE REACTIONS

–D/C drug immediately and initiate appropriate treatment for symptoms.

–Treat insulin shock with 50% dextrose IV.
–Treat diabetic coma (DKA) with insulin SC and IV until desired results.

OTHER REACTIONS

–Notify physician of any side effects; initiate appropriate actions.

IPECAC SYRUP Ipecac

CLASS

–Emetic

USES

–Induce vomiting in poisoning

ACTION

–Irritates gastric mucosa and stimulates chemoreceptor trigger zone for emesis

USUAL DOSAGE/ROUTE

ADULT

–PO: 15 ml followed by 100–200 ml water

PEDIATRIC

–PO (children at least 1 yr): 15 ml followed by 100–200 ml water
–PO (children less than 1 yr): 5–10 ml followed by 100–200 ml water, may repeat in 20 min as needed

ADVERSE/SIDE EFFECTS

RAPID

–NVD
–Sedation
–Dysrhythmias
–Circulatory failure
–Convulsions
–Coma

GRADUAL

–Depression
–Bloody diarrhea

CONTRAINDICATIONS

–Hypersensitivity
–Depressed gag reflex
–Poisoning with petroleum products or caustic substance (Lye, Drano)
–Convulsions

SPECIAL PRECAUTIONS

–Pregnant or lactating patients
–Children less than 6 mo old, safety not established

OTHER SPECIAL INFORMATION

–Do not confuse syrup with fluid extract, which is 14 times stronger.
–Drug effectiveness is reduced if given with milk or carbonated beverage.
–Bounce child to increase emetic effects.
–Monitor vital signs, especially respirations after drug ingestion.
–Patient must have emesis before activated charcoal can be given effectively.

ANTIDOTE

SEVERE REACTIONS

–D/C drug immediately and initiate appropriate treatment for symptoms.

OTHER REACTIONS

–Notify physician of any side effects and initiate appropriate actions.
–If patient does not vomit in 10–15 mins, give ACTIVATED CHARCOAL and lavage the stomach.

IRON DEXTRAN INJECTION Dextraron, Feostat, Imferon, K-Feron, Nor-feron, and others

CLASS
–Iron preparation

USES
–Iron deficiency anemia when oral iron preparations are not adequately therapeutic or possible
–Severe anemia where hemoglobin less than 7.5 gm/dl (normal male = 13.5–18 gm/dl; female = 12–16 gm/dl)

ACTION
–Slow absorption into reticuloendothelial system where ferric iron is transported by transferrin and incorporated into hemoglobin in the bone marrow

USUAL DOSAGE/ROUTE
ADULT (over 60 kg)
–IM: 50 mg first day, and up to 250 mg every other day or twice weekly
–IV: 15–30 mg first day, increasing by 10 mg daily until hemoglobin levels return to normal

ADULT AND PEDIATRIC (9–59 kg)
–No more than 100 mg IM daily

INFANTS (3.5–9 kg)
–No more than 50 mg IM daily

INFANTS (under 3.5 kg)
–No more than 25 mg IM daily

ADVERSE/SIDE EFFECTS
RAPID
–Possible anaphylactic reaction
–Dyspnea
–Hypotension

–N & V
–Metallic taste
–Shivering
–Seizures
–Rash, pruritis, urticaria
–Shock
–Tachycardia
–Leukocytosis

GRADUAL
–Phlebitis
–Febrile episodes
–Soreness, inflammation, or abscess at or near injection site
–Brown skin discoloration at injection site
–Leukocytosis

CONTRAINDICATIONS
–Hypersensitivity to Imferon
–In all anemias other than iron deficiency anemia
–Hepatic disease

SPECIAL PRECAUTIONS
–Pregnant or lactating patients
–Acute renal disease
–Asthma
–Rheumatoid arthritis
–Children and infants less than 4 months

OTHER SPECIAL INFORMATION
–Use Z-track method of IM injection to prevent tissue damage and skin discoloration at injection site.
–Inject medication into buttock deeply with 2-inch 18–19 gauge needle.
–Alternate injection sites.
–Do not mix with other drugs or D_5W.
–Administer a test dose of 25 mg by preferred route at least 1 hr before starting therapy to assess for reactions.

ANTIDOTE

SEVERE REACTIONS

–D/C drug immediately and initiate appropriate treatment for symptoms.

–Treat iron overdose (poisoning) with DEFEROXAMINE (Desferol), which is a chelating agent.

OTHER REACTIONS

–Notify physician of any side effects and initiate appropriate actions.

ISOPROTERENOL HCL, ISOPROTERENOL SULFATE **Aerolone, Isuprel, Medihaler-Iso, Proternol, Vapo-Iso, and others**

CLASS

–Beta-adrenergic, antidysrhythmic, bronchodilator

USES

–Bronchodilator in reversible airway obstruction due to asthma, COPD, or bronchospasm

–Management of ventricular dysrhythmias, Adams-Stokes syndrome, heart blocks

–Treatment of shock associated with decreased cardiac output and vasoconstriction

ACTION

–Relaxes smooth muscle of bronchi (beta-2)

–Positive inotropic and chronotropic actions increase cardiac output by increasing force of contraction and increase venous return to heart

–Cardiac stimulant that increases rate of contraction (beta-1)

–Lowers peripheral vascular resistance

USUAL DOSAGE/ROUTE

ADULT

–*Bronchospasm:* SL: 10–20 mg not to exceed 60 mg/day

–*Heart block ventricular dysrhythmias:* SL: 10–15 mg 4–6 times/day; IM: 0.2 mg, then 0.02–1 mg as needed; IV: 0.02–0.06 mg, then 2–10 mcg/min as needed

PEDIATRIC

–*Bronchospasm:* SL: 5–10 mg not to exceed 30 mg/day

–*Heart block:* SL: 5–12.5 mg 4–6 times/day; IM: 0.1 mg, then 0.01–0.5 mg as needed; IV: 0.01–0.03 mg, then 1–5 mcg/min as needed

ADULT AND PEDIATRIC

–*Asthma, bronchitis:* 1–5 inhalation treatments as needed daily

–*Shock:* IV: Infuse 0.5–5 mcg/min (1 mg in 500 ml D_5W) adjusted according to heart rate, BP, and urine output

ADVERSE/SIDE EFFECTS

RAPID

–Cardiac arrest
–Hypotension
–Increased myocardial oxygen consumption and work (tachycardia)
–Angina-type pain
–Palpitations
–Sweating
–Hyperglycemia
–Anxiety
–Tremors

GRADUAL

–Insomnia
–Headache
–N & V

CONTRAINDICATIONS

–Hypersensitivity to the drug
–Preexisting cardiac dysrhythmias
–Narrow-angle glaucoma

SPECIAL PRECAUTIONS
–Pregnant or lactating patients
–Cardiac disorders
–Hyperthyroidism
–Prostatic hypertrophy
–Elderly

OTHER SPECIAL INFORMATION
–Do not use with MAO inhibitors.
–Avoid use of this drug with EPINEPHRINE, PROPRANOLOL, or tricyclic antidepressants, such as NORPRAMINE, SINEQUAN.
–Monitor patient for respiratory problems.
–Patient's saliva may appear pink after inhalation therapy.
–Newer beta-specific and longer-acting agents should be used in asthma.

ANTIDOTE

SEVERE REACTIONS
–D/C drug immediately and initiate appropriate treatment for symptoms.
–Treat overdose with a beta-blocker such as PROPRANOLOL ATENOLOL, TIMOLOL, or METOPROLOL.

OTHER REACTIONS
–Notify physician of any side effects and initiate appropriate actions.

ISOSORBIDE DINITRATE Isordil, Iso-bid, Isorbid, Sorbitrate, and others

CLASS
–Nitrate antianginal, smooth muscle relaxant

USES
–Prophylactically to decrease frequency of coronary insufficiency and angina pectoris

ACTION

–Mechanism of action causes venous pooling in extremities and decreases cardiac work by decreasing preload and afterload; relaxes smooth muscle

USUAL DOSAGE/ROUTE

ADULT

–SL: 2.5–10 mg every 2–3 hr as needed
–Chewable tab: 5 mg initially, then lowest effective dosage 4 times/day
–PO dosing: 10–30 mg 3–4 times/day initially, working up to 50–60 mg every 4–6 hr

PEDIATRIC

–Safe use in children not established

ADVERSE/SIDE EFFECTS

RAPID

–Hypotension
–Tachycardia
–Cutaneous vasodilation with flushing
–Headache
–Flushing
–Dizziness
–Transient weakness or dizziness

GRADUAL

–Postural hypotension
–N & V

CONTRAINDICATIONS

–Hypersensitivity to this drug or other nitrites
–Severe anemia
–Increased intracranial pressure
–Acute MI
–Cerebral hemorrhage

SPECIAL PRECAUTIONS

–Pregnant or lactating patients
–Postural hypotension

–Head trauma
–Children

OTHER SPECIAL INFORMATION

–Administer with meals to prevent or reduce headaches.
–Instruct patient not to swallow sublingual tablets.
–PO onset = 15–30 min; duration = 4–6 hr.
–SL onset = 2–5 min; duration = 1–2 hr.
–Chewable tab onset = 3 min; duration = ½–3 hr.
–If 3 SL tabs in 15 mins does not relieve pain, go to the emergency department.

ANTIDOTE

SEVERE REACTIONS

–D/C drug immediately and initiate appropriate treatment for symptoms.

OTHER REACTIONS

–Notify physician of any side effects and initiate appropriate actions.

ISOXSUPRINE HCL Vasodilan, Voxsuprine

CLASS

–Peripheral vasodilator

USES

–Cerebrovascular insufficiency

ACTION

–Increases blood flow by acting on vascular smooth muscle
–Causes uterine relaxation and cardiac stimulation

USUAL DOSAGE/ROUTE

ADULT

–PO: 10–20 mg 3–4 times daily

PEDIATRIC
–Safe use in children not established

ADVERSE/SIDE EFFECTS

RAPID
–Tachycardia
–Hypotension

GRADUAL
–Rash
–Flushing
–Dizziness
–N & V

CONTRAINDICATIONS

–Hypersensitivity
–Postpartum use

SPECIAL PRECAUTIONS

–Use in pregnancy
–Tachycardia

OTHER SPECIAL INFORMATION

–Take with food to avoid GI upset.
–Avoid use in persons who smoke; will cause added vasoconstriction.
–Peak = 1 hr; half life = 1¼ hr; duration = 3 hr.
–This drug does cross placenta and will effect the fetus.

ANTIDOTE

SEVERE REACTIONS
–D/C drug immediately and initiate appropriate treatment for symptoms.

OTHER REACTIONS
–Notify physician of any side effects and initiate appropriate actions.

KETOROLAC Toradol

CLASS
–Nonsteroidal anti-inflammatory, antipyretic, analgesic

USES
–Mild-to-moderate pain
–Osteoarthritis
–Rheumatoid arthritis

ACTION
–Inhibits prostaglandin synthesis by decreasing an enzyme needed for biosynthesis

USUAL DOSAGE/ROUTE
ADULT
–IM: 30–60 mg loading dose, then 15–30 mg every 6 hr

PEDIATRIC
–Safe use in children not established

ADVERSE/SIDE EFFECTS
RAPID
–Dizziness
–Drowsiness
–N & V
–Tachycardia

GRADUAL
–GI tract ulceration/bleeding
–Peripheral edema
–Constipation
–Flatulence
–Nephrotoxicity
–Ototoxicity
–Oliguria
–Blood dyscrasia
–Insomnia

CONTRAINDICATIONS
–Hypersensitivity to this drug and other anti-inflammatory agents
–Asthma
–Renal disease
–Hepatic disease

SPECIAL PRECAUTIONS
–Pregnant or lactating patients
–Children
–Bleeding disorders
–Cardiac disorders

OTHER SPECIAL INFORMATION
–Action of drug increased by KETOROLAC, PHENYTOIN, SULFONAMIDES.
–Monitor hepatic and renal function.
–Give with food to reduce GI upset.

ANTIDOTE

SEVERE REACTIONS
–D/C drug immediately and initiate appropriate treatment for symptoms.

OTHER REACTIONS
–Notify physician of any side effects and initiate appropriate actions.

LABETALOL Normodyne, Trandate

CLASS
–Beta-adrenergic blocker (antihypertensive)

USES
–Hypertension
–Angina

ACTION
–Stimulation of beta-1 and beta-2 receptor sites, causing peripheral vasodilation, orthostatic hypotension, and decreased heart rate and blood pressure

USUAL DOSAGE/ROUTE
ADULT
–PO: 100 mg 2 times/day, and increase by 100 mg 2 times/day every 2–3 days until BP controlled, then maintenance 200–400 mg 2 times/day
–IV: 20 mg then 40–80 mg at 2 mg/min at 10-min intervals (max 300 mg total dose)

PEDIATRIC
–Safe use in children not established

ADVERSE/SIDE EFFECTS
RAPID
–Orthostatic hypotension
–Weakness
–Bradycardia
–Bronchospasm

GRADUAL
–Fatigue
–CHF
–Pulmonary edema
–Rash
–Hypoglycemia or hyperglycemia
–Joint pain

CONTRAINDICATIONS
–Hypersensitivity
–Uncompensated CHF
–Cardiogenic shock
–Bradycardia
–Pregnancy, lactation

SPECIAL PRECAUTIONS
–Thyrotoxicosis
–Hypoglycemia
–Renal impairment (may take reduced dosage)

OTHER SPECIAL INFORMATION
–Do not withdraw drug abruptly.
–Effects of drug may increase if given with HALOTHANE, cardiac glycosides, other antihypertensive agents, nitrates, alcohol.
–Toxicity may occur if given with CIMETIDINE.
–This drug is absorbed better if taken with food.
–Do not give if pulse less than 50 beats/min.

ANTIDOTE

SEVERE REACTIONS
–D/C drug immediately and initiate appropriate treatment for symptoms.

OTHER REACTIONS
–Notify physician of any side effects and initiate appropriate actions.

LIDOCAINE HCL INTRAVENOUS Lidocaine, Xylocaine

CLASS
–Antidysrhythmic

USES

–Treatment of acute ventricular dysrhythmias (PVCs, tachycardia, fibrillation) occurring during a myocardial infarction or during surgical procedures such as cardiac catheterization

ACTION

–Shortens the refractory period and suppresses the ventricular automaticity of ectopic foci during diastole

USUAL DOSAGE/ROUTE

ADULT

–IV bolus: 50–100 mg at a rate of 25–50 mg/min and may repeat at 5-min intervals up to 300 mg (onset = 10 sec)
–IV infusion: 1–4 mg/min (suggested dilution 2 gm in 500 ml dextrose solution (equals 4 mg/ml) (onset = 10–20 min)
–IM: 4.3 mg/kg up to 300 mg and may repeat after 60–90 min
–Maximum dose: 200–300 mg in 1 hr period

PEDIATRIC

–IV bolus: 0.5–1.0 mg/kg up to 15–25 mg and may repeat at 5-min intervals up to 3 mg/kg
–IV infusion: 0.01–0.05 mg/kg/min up to a maximum of 5 mg/kg (suggested dilution of 1 gm in 500 ml dextrose solution equals 2 mg/ml) (onset = 10–20 min)

ADVERSE/SIDE EFFECTS

RAPID

–Hypotension
–Bradycardia
–Cardiac arrest

GRADUAL

–N & V
–Anxiety
–Widening of QRS complex
–Convulsions
–Respiratory depression and arrest

–Dizziness, drowsiness
–Sensations of heat, cold, or numbness
–Blurred vision
–Tinnitus

CONTRAINDICATIONS
–Hypersensitivity to drug
–Stokes–Adams syndrome
–Wolff–Parkinson–White syndrome
–Severe SA, AV, or intraventricular block
–PVCs in conjunction with bradycardia

SPECIAL PRECAUTIONS
–Pregnant or lactating patients
–Liver or kidney disease (decrease dosage)
–Congestive heart failure (decrease dosage)

OTHER SPECIAL INFORMATION
–Monitor ECG frequently.
–Have resuscitative equipment available.
–Use IV infusion controller when administering IV infusion.
–Monitor patient for CNS effects.
–Observe vital signs at least every hour.
–Taper dosage after 24 hr of continuous therapy.

ANTIDOTE
SEVERE REACTIONS
–D/C drug immediately and initiate appropriate treatment for symptoms.
–Treat anaphylactic shock with EPINEPHRINE HCL and corticosteroids such as METHYLPREDNISOLONE.
–Treat CNS stimulation with antianxiety drugs such as DIAZEPAM, rapid short-acting barbiturates such as PENTOBARBITAL, or short-acting muscle relaxants such as SUCCINYL CHOLINE.
–Treat hypotension with vasopressors such as DOPAMINE.

OTHER REACTIONS
–Notify physician of any side effects and initiate appropriate actions.

LIDOCAINE HCL LOCAL, LIDOCAINE HCL WITH EPINEPHRINE LOCAL **Ardecaine, L-Caine E, Nervocaine, Norocaine, Xylocaine, Xylocaine Topical, and others**

CLASS
–Local anesthetic

USES
–Nerve block (peripheral, sympathetic, central)
–Spinal, caudal, epidural anesthesia
–Surface anesthesia of skin and mucous membranes

ACTION
–Local anesthetics stabilize the neuronal membrane by decreasing its ion permeability, thereby preventing initiation and conduction of nerve impulses
–Use of LIDOCAINE with EPINEPHRINE (a vasoconstrictor) prolongs the duration of action by decreasing systemic absorption

USUAL DOSAGE/ROUTE

ADULT AND PEDIATRIC
–Dosage varies and depends upon the area to be anesthetized, the vascularity of the tissues, the neuronal segments to be blocked, individual tolerance, and the technique of anesthesia.
–The smallest dosage producing effective anesthesia should be used.

ADVERSE/SIDE EFFECTS

RAPID
–Hypersensitivity characterized by urticaria, edema, or anaphylaxis
–Loss of consciousness
–Tremors
–Shivering

–Pupil constriction
–Blurred vision
–Convulsions
–N & V
–Status asthmaticus
–Respiratory depression/arrest
–Cardiac arrest
–Hypotension
–Bradycardia
–Dysrhythmias
–Paresthesias
–Pupil constriction

CONTRAINDICATIONS
–Hypersensitivity to local anesthetics
–Severe liver disease
–Use of local anesthetics with vasopressors in the presence of oxytoxic drugs
–Preparations containing preservatives should not be used for spinal or epidural anesthesia

SPECIAL PRECAUTIONS
–Elderly
–Children under 12 years
–Pregnant patients
–Drug allergies
–Liver disease

OTHER SPECIAL INFORMATION
–Duration of action is 1–1½ hours, with rapid metabolism of the drug occurring in the liver.
–Use LIDOCAINE with EPINEPHRINE with extreme caution in persons receiving known MAO inhibitors, tricyclic antidepressants, and phenothiazines, because severe hypotension or hypertension may result.
–LIDOCAINE with EPINEPHRINE may produce severe dysrhythmias when used in patients during or following the administration of CHLOROFORM, HALOTHANE, CYCLOPROPANE, TRICHLOROETHYLENE.

–All solutions of this drug without preservatives should be discarded after initial use.
–Avoid IV injection; use a slow rate of injection to reduce systemic reaction.
–Use LIDOCAINE with EPINEPHRINE cautiously in areas of compromised blood supply (nose, ears, fingers, toes) or in the presence of peripheral vascular disease to prevent exaggerated vasoconstriction response.
–Oral topical anesthetics may interfere with swallowing; do not give patient food or fluid at least 60 minutes after drug application and until gag reflex returns.

ANTIDOTE

SEVERE REACTIONS

–D/C drug immediately and initiate appropriate treatment for symptoms.
–In cardiac respiratory arrest, initiate ALS procedures as indicated including oxygen & IV fluids.
–Treat seizures with anticonvulsants.
–Treat hypotension with vasopressors such as DOPAMINE or NOREPINEPHRINE.

OTHER REACTIONS

–Notify physician of any side effects and initiate appropriate actions.

LISINOPRIL Prinivil, Zestril

CLASS

–Angiotensin-converting enzyme (ACE) inhibitor (antihypertensive)

USES

–Mild-to-moderate hypertension

ACTION

–Inhibits angiotensin-converting enzyme conversion of angiotensin I to angiotensin II, decreasing arterial and venous vasoconstriction and reducing sodium retention

USUAL DOSAGE/ROUTE

ADULT

–PO: 10–40 mg/day increasing up to 80 mg/day to desired effect (decreasing dose to half with concurrent use of diuretics)

PEDIATRIC

–Safe use in children not established

ADVERSE/SIDE EFFECTS

RAPID

–Hypotension
–NVD
–Rash/pruritus
–Vertigo
–Bronchospasm/laryngospasm
–Dyspnea/cough
–Fever/chills
–Paresthesias

GRADUAL

–Anorexia
–Constipation
–GI irritation
–Proteinuria
–Renal insufficiency
–Impotence
–Depression
–Insomnia
–Dizziness/light-headedness
–Altered taste
–Hyperkalemia
–Neutropenia
–Headache
–Fatigue

–Weakness
–Stomatitis

CONTRAINDICATIONS
–Hypersensitivity
–Pregnant or lactating patients
–Heart block
–In conjunction with potassium-sparing diuretics
–Children

SPECIAL PRECAUTIONS
–Renal disease
–Thyroid disease
–COPD
–Asthma
–Dialysis patients
–Hypovolemia
–Hyperkalemia
–Diabetes mellitus

OTHER SPECIAL INFORMATION
–PO onset = 1 hr; peak = 6–8 hr; duration = 24 hr.
–Aspirin and INDOMETHACIN decrease the effect of this drug.
–Use with extreme caution in renal dysfunction.
–Do not give with potassium supplements, potassium-sparing diuretics, or with vasodilators.
–Monitor BP frequently for decreases during use.
–This drug may cause proteinuria.

ANTIDOTE
SEVERE REACTIONS
–D/C drug immediately and initiate appropriate treatment for symptoms.
–Lavage stomach.
–Expand fluid volume with NS and place in supine or Trendelenburg position for severe hypotension.
–Treat bradycardia with IV ATROPINE.
–Treat bronchospasm/laryngospasm with IV THEOPHYLLINE and OXYGEN.

–Treat cardiac failure with diuretics.
–Treat severe reactions with hemodialysis.

OTHER REACTIONS

–Notify physician of any side effects and initiate appropriate actions.

LORAZEPAM Alzapam, Ativan, Loraz

CLASS

–Sedative/hypnotic (antianxiety)

USES

–Preanesthesia medication
–Sedation for insomnia
–Anxiety, tension, agitation, irritability
–Anticonvulsant
–Alcohol withdrawal symptoms.

ACTION

–Depresses subcortical levels of CNS

USUAL DOSAGE/ROUTE

ADULT

–PO: 2–10 mg/day in divided doses with a larger dose at bedtime
–IM: 2–4 mg up to a maximum of 4 mg
–IV: 2–4 mg
–IV preoperative: 1–12 mg or 50 mcg/kg IM or IV

PEDIATRIC

–Not commonly administered in children younger than 18 years

ADVERSE/SIDE EFFECTS

RAPID

–Dizziness
–Restlessness

–Crying
–Burning at administration site with IM and IV use
–N & V
–Rash
–Orthostatic hypotension
–Tachycardia
–Blurred vision

GRADUAL
–Depression
–Fatigue
–Insomnia
–Constipation
–Anorexia

CONTRAINDICATIONS
–Hypersensitivity
–Pregnancy: may cause fetal damage
–Psychosis
–Acute narrow-angle glaucoma
–Children under 12 years
–Asthma
–COPD
–History of drug abuse

SPECIAL PRECAUTIONS
–Elderly (reduced dosage)
–Debilitated
–Liver disease
–Renal disease

OTHER SPECIAL INFORMATION
–When given IV, mix ½ strength with diluent and do not exceed 2 mg/min IV rate of infusion.
–Partial airway obstruction with oversedation is possible.
–Steady state is reached after 2–3 days.
–Pharmacologic mechanism is similar to DIAZEPAM (Valium).

ANTIDOTE

SEVERE REACTIONS

–D/C drug immediately and initiate appropriate treatment for symptoms.

–Treat overdose with gastric lavage and frequent monitoring of VS.

OTHER REACTIONS

–Notify physician of any side effects and initiate appropriate actions.

MAGNESIUM SULFATE Bilagog, Epsom Salt

CLASS

–Anticonvulsant, electrolyte, saline laxative

USES

–Anticonvulsant in seizures associated with tetanus, eclampsia, glomerulonephritis, hypothyroidism, and hypomagnesemia
–Cathartic to relieve acute constipation, reduces edema and ascites and rids intestinal tract of food and drug poisons
–Cerebral edema
–Antidote for barium poisoning

ACTION

–Parenteral administration depresses central nervous system and smooth, skeletal, and cardiac muscle.
–Unabsorbed salts use osmotic action to draw water into intestines; peristalsis is increased, thereby decreasing absorption of fluids from the bowel.

USUAL DOSAGE/ROUTE

ADULT

–*Laxative:* PO: 10–30 gm
–*Anticonvulsant:* IM: 1–5 gm in 25–50% solution; IV: 1–4 gm in 10–20% solution, or infuse 4 gm in 250 ml of D_5W
–*Magnesium deficiency:* IM or IV: 1 gm every 6 hours, up to 250 mg/kg for severe deficiencies
–*Barium poisoning:* IV: 1–2 gm
–*Cerebral edema:* IV: up to 2.5 gm

PEDIATRIC

–*Laxative:* PO: 6–12 yr, 5–10 gm; 2–5 yr, 2.5–5 gm
–*Anticonvulsant:* IV: 20–40 mg/kg in a 20% solution, repeated as needed
–*Barium poisoning:* IV: 1–2 gm
–*Cerebral edema:* IV: up to 2.5 gm

ADVERSE/SIDE EFFECTS

RAPID

- –Sweating
- –Flushing
- –Respiratory and circulatory collapse
- –Hypotension
- –Sedation
- –Flaccid paralysis
- –Heart block

GRADUAL

- –Hypermagnesemia
- –Depressed reflexes
- –Weakness
- –Hypothermia
- –Decreased cardiac function

CONTRAINDICATIONS

- –Hypersensitivity
- –Hypermagnesemia
- –Bowel obstruction
- –Hemorrhage
- –Myocardial infarction
- –Inflammatory disorder of GI tract
- –Renal disease

SPECIAL PRECAUTIONS

- –Mental depression
- –Pregnant patients
- –Heart block

OTHER SPECIAL INFORMATION

- –For laxative action, drug is best taken before breakfast with plenty of water or fruit juice.
- –Ice chips or flavoring such as lemon juice reduce the unpleasant taste of this drug.
- –Monitor intake and output for possible dehydration.
- –Patients receiving parenteral drug should be constantly attended; vital signs should be taken every 10–15 min.
- –Administer IM drug in deep gluteal sites.

–Watch for respiratory depression.
–This may be best drug to use in early alcoholic withdrawal (600 mg 4 times/day).

ANTIDOTE

SEVERE REACTIONS
–D/C drug immediately and initiate appropriate treatment for symptoms.
–Antidote for this drug is CALCIUM GLUCONATE.

OTHER REACTIONS
–Notify physician of any side effects and initiate appropriate actions.

MANNITOL Mannitol

CLASS
–Osmotic diuretic

USES
–Evaluation of glomerular filtration rate
–Prevention or treatment of oliguria secondary to renal insufficiency
–Reduction of intracranial pressure and cerebral edema (within 15 min)
–Promotion of urinary secretion of toxic secretions
–Diuresis in drug intoxication

ACTION
–Increases the osmolarity of the blood to draw fluid from the intracellular and extracellular spaces
–Prevents reabsorption of water in the renal tubules
–Acts within 30–60 min on acute narrow-angle glaucoma, either absolute or secondary

USUAL DOSAGE/ROUTE

ADULT

–*Oliguria:* IV: 50–200 gm of a 5%, 10%, 15% solution over 24 hr adjusted to maintain urine output of 30–50 ml/hr

–*Test dose:* 200 mg/kg (or 12.5 gm) given IV over 3–5 min; if increase in urine output after 5 min, the full dose by infusion can be given

–*Increased intracranial or intraocular pressure:* IV: 1.5–2.0 gm/kg over 30–60 min of a 15–20% solution

–*Excretion of toxic substances:* IV: Up to 200 gm over 30–60 min of a 5–10% solution repeated until blood levels of substance show clearance

–*Elevation of glomerular filtration:* IV: 100 ml of 20% solution added to 180 ml NS infused over 30 min

PEDIATRIC (over 12 yr)

–*Oliguria:* IV: 2 g/kg as 15–20% solution over 2–6 hr

–*Increased intracranial or intraocular pressure:* IV: 2 g/kg as 15–20% solution over 30–60 min

–*Excretion of toxic substances:* IV: 2 g/kg as 5–10% solution over 30–60 min

ADVERSE/SIDE EFFECTS

RAPID

–Circulatory overload
–Pulmonary edema
–Water intoxication with rapid infusion
–Convulsions
–Dizziness
–Chest pain
–NVD
–Hypo- and hypertension
–Hypo- and hyperkalemia
–Hypo- and hypernatremia

GRADUAL

–Headache
–Thirst
–Fever
–Chills

–Dehydration
–Electrolyte loss
–Loss of hearing
–Decreased intraocular pressure

CONTRAINDICATIONS
–Hypersensitivity
–Well-established anuria due to renal disease
–Failure to respond to test dose in 3–5 min
–Dehydration
–Active intracranial bleeding

SPECIAL PRECAUTIONS
–Pregnant or lactating patients
–Severe renal disease
–CHF, PE

OTHER SPECIAL INFORMATION
–Monitor serum sodium and potassium levels.
–Do not mix with potassium chloride, blood, or CEPHALOSPORINS.
–Avoid extravasation (local edema, skin necrosis).
–Monitor renal function frequently during use (BUN, creatinine, hydration, urine-specific gravity).
–Administer IV undiluted and use an inline filter.
–If IV solution contains crystals, warm bottle in hot water and shake vigorously.
–Monitor neurologic status, visual acuity.

ANTIDOTE

SEVERE REACTIONS
–D/C drug immediately and initiate appropriate treatment for symptoms.

OTHER REACTIONS
–Notify physician of any side effects and initiate appropriate actions.

MECAMYLAMINE HCL Inversine

CLASS
–Antihypertensive (ganglionic blocking agent)

USES
–Moderate-to-severe essential hypertension
–Uncomplicated malignant hypertension

ACTION
–Competes with acetylcholine by blocking transmission of impulses at the sympathetic and parasympathetic ganglia, causing vasodilation and lowered blood pressure

USUAL DOSAGE/ROUTE
ADULT
–PO: 2.5 mg 2 times/day initially, increasing or decreasing in increments of 2.5 mg/day every 2–3 days until desired BP is achieved; maintenance dose is 25 mg/day in 2–4 divided doses

PEDIATRIC
–Safe use in children not established

ADVERSE/SIDE EFFECTS
RAPID
–N & V
–Convulsions
–Tremors
–Paresthesias
–Dizziness
–Syncope
–Postural hypotension
–Dilated pupils
–Blurred vision
–Tachycardia

GRADUAL
–Hypotension
–Mental aberrations

–Glossitis
–Dry mouth
–Constipation
–Anorexia
–Urinary retention and dysuria
–Paralytic ileus
–Sexual dysfunction

CONTRAINDICATIONS
–Hypersensitivity
–Pregnant or lactating patients
–Coronary insufficiency
–History of recent myocardial infarction
–Uremia
–Glaucoma
–Pyloric stenosis
–Chronic pyelonephritis
–In conjunction with sulfonamides

SPECIAL PRECAUTIONS
–Coronary atherosclerosis
–Cerebral atherosclerosis
–History of recent CVA
–Renal insufficiency (prolongs excretion up to 24 hr)
–Sodium restriction (enhances effects)
–Prostatic hypertrophy
–Bladder neck obstruction
–Urethral stricture

OTHER SPECIAL INFORMATION
–Antihypertensive effects begins in ½–2 hr, and peak = 3–5 hr.
–This drug does elicit anticholinergic effects and may exacerbate urinary obstructive disorders.
–This drug should not be discontinued abruptly; severe rebound hypertension can occur.

ANTIDOTE

SEVERE REACTIONS

–D/C drug immediately and initiate appropriate treatment for symptoms.

–Treat overdose with gastric lavage and give activated charcoal, then treat symptomatically.

–Treat hypotension with small doses of a vasopressor such as DOPAMINE.

OTHER REACTIONS

–Notify physician of any side effects and initiate appropriate actions.

MEPERIDINE HCL Demerol, Pethidine

CLASS

–Narcotic analgesic (opiate derivative)

USES

–For relief of moderate-to-severe pain

–A preoperative and postoperative medicine

–For support of anesthesia

ACTION

–Interferes with pain impulses at the subcortical level on the brain to produce sedation, analgesia, and euphoria

–Increases gastrointestinal smooth muscle tone

USUAL DOSAGE/ROUTE

ADULT

–PO, SC, IM, IV: 50–150 mg every 3–4 hr as needed

–*Preoperative:* IM: 50–100 mg 30–90 min before anesthesia

PEDIATRIC

–PO, SC, IM: 1 mg/kg every 4–6 hr as needed to a maximum of 100 mg every 4 hr

–*Preoperative* (over 1 year): SC, IM: 1.0–2.0 mg/kg 30–90 minutes before anesthesia; (less than 1 year): no narcotic, just ATROPINE 0.01 mg/kg IM

ADVERSE/SIDE EFFECTS

RAPID

–N & V
–Drowsiness
–Dizziness
–Respiratory depression
–Orthostatic hypotension
–Confusion
–Headache
–Sedation
–Euphoria
–Increased intracranial pressure
–Rash
–Palpitations
–Bradycardia
–Tachycardia (IV use)

GRADUAL

–Constipation
–Anorexia
–GI cramps
–Urinary retention
–Dysuria
–Diaphoresis
–Depression of cough reflex

CONTRAINDICATIONS

–Hypersensitivity
–Patients who have received MAO inhibitors (antidepressants) in the past 2 weeks
–Increased intracranial pressure (loss of pupillary reflex)
–Pregnancy, before labor

SPECIAL PRECAUTIONS

–Addictive personality
–Pregnant or lactating patients

–MI patients
–Respiratory depression
–Liver disease
–Renal disease
–Children less than 18 years

OTHER SPECIAL INFORMATION

–Monitor respiratory status, especially in COPD and asthma patients.
–For IV administration, dilute 1 mg/1 cc of D_5W or NS and infuse very slowly.
–There are potentiated effects if used concurrently with HYDROXYZINE.
–Patient must be lying down during and after administration because of CNS depression and orthostatic hypotension potential.
–NORMEPERIDINE (a metabolite) may precipitate seizures in epileptic patients.
–NORMEPERIDINE will accumulate in sickle cell anemia patients, producing toxic reactions.
–PO absorption is erratic and unreliable.
–Use in reduced doses and with caution in patients with myxedema, Addison's disease, and hepatic cirrhosis.

ANTIDOTE

SEVERE REACTIONS

–D/C drug immediately and initiate appropriate treatment for symptoms.
–Treat overdose with NALOXONE 0.2–0.8 mg IV, OXYGEN, IV fluids, and vasopressors such as DOPAMINE.

OTHER REACTIONS

–Notify physician of any side effects and initiate appropriate actions.

METAPROTERENOL SULFATE Alupent, Metaprel

CLASS
–Beta-2 adrenergic (bronchodilator)

USES
–Bronchial asthma
–Decrease bronchospasms associated with bronchitis and emphysema

ACTION
–Relaxes bronchial smooth muscle by direct action on the beta-2 adrenergic receptors

USUAL DOSAGE/ROUTE
ADULT AND PEDIATRIC (over 12 yr)
–PO: 20 mg 3–4 times/day
–Inhaler: 2–3 inhalations 3–4 times/day not to exceed 12 treatments in 24 hr

PEDIATRIC (under 12 yr)
–Age 9–12 yr: 20 mg PO 3–4 times/day
–Age 6–9 yr: 10 mg PO 3–4 times/day
–PO not recommended for children under age 6
–Inhaler not recommended for children under age 12

ADVERSE/SIDE EFFECTS
RAPID
–Tachycardia
–Palpitations
–Hypertension
–Dysrhythmias
–Tremors
–Anxiety
–Headache
–Cardiac arrest
–Dyspnea

GRADUAL
–Nervousness
–N & V
–Insomnia
–Hyperglycemia

CONTRAINDICATIONS
–Hypersensitivity
–Children under 6 yr
–Patients with cardiac dysrhythmias associated with tachycardia

SPECIAL PRECAUTIONS
–Pregnant patients
–Cardiac disorders
–Hyperthyroidism
–Diabetes mellitus
–Prostatic hypertrophy

OTHER SPECIAL INFORMATION
–PO onset = 15–30 min; peak = 1 hr; duration = 4 hr.
–Administer 2 hr before bedtime to avoid sleeplessness.
–During acute bronchospasm, dose using sequential step inhalation; e.g., 1 puff, hold breath for 10 seconds, repeat 1 puff, hold for 10 seconds, repeat 2- puff cycle 3 times in 15–20 min.

ANTIDOTE

SEVERE REACTIONS
–D/C drug immediately and initiate appropriate treatment for symptoms.

OTHER REACTIONS
–Notify physician of any side effects and initiate appropriate actions.

METARAMINOL BITARTRATE Aramine

CLASS
–Adrenergic agent (vasopressor)

USES
–Hypotension
–Shock

ACTION
–Increases blood pressure through vasoconstriction
–Inhibits GI, smooth skeletal muscle
–Increases heart rate, force of contraction
–Reduces perfusion to vital organs

USUAL DOSAGE/ROUTE

ADULT
–IM, SC: 2–10 mg not repeated for 10 min
–IV: 0.5 mg over 1 min followed by continuous infusion
–IV infusion: 15–100 mg in 500 ml solution (Dextrose, Normal Saline, Ringer); rate titrated to achieve and maintain blood pressure desired

PEDIATRIC
–IM, SC: 0.1 mg/kg not repeated for 10 min
–IV: 0.4 mg/kg diluted and infused to achieve and maintain desired BP

ADVERSE/SIDE EFFECTS

RAPID
–Dysrhythmias
–Cardiac arrest
–Headache
–Hypertension
–Convulsions
–Palpitations
–Angina

GRADUAL

–Local tissue sloughing from necrosis of site tissue
–N&V
–Apprehension, anxiety
–Flushing, pallor

CONTRAINDICATIONS

–Hypersensitivity to METARAMINOLS, PARABENS, BISULFITES
–Peripheral or mesenteric vascular disease
–Hypoxia
–Hypercapnia
–Pheochromocytoma

SPECIAL PRECAUTIONS

–Pregnant or lactating patients
–Hypertension, hyperthyroidism, heart disease, diabetes mellitus, liver disease, peripheral vascular disease

OTHER SPECIAL INFORMATION

–Monitor injection/infusion site for tissue necrosis.
–Drug action increased if given with ATROPINE, beta-adrenergic blockers.
–Drug action reduced if given with diuretics, alpha-adrenergic blockers.
–Monitor BP and urine output frequently with therapy.
–Onset of action IV: 1–2 min, IM/SC: 10 min; duration IM, SC, IV: 20 min–1 hr.

ANTIDOTE

SEVERE REACTIONS

–D/C drug immediately and initiate appropriate treatment for symptoms.
–Administer alpha-blocker such as PRAZOSIN, HYTRIN, then NOREPINEPHRINE.

METHYLDOPA HCL, METHYLDOPATE
Aldomet, Dopamet, Medimet, Novomedopa

CLASS
–Antihypertensive (adrenergic inhibitor)

USES
–Moderate-to-severe hypertension

ACTION
–Depresses activity of sympathetic nervous system
–Decreases arterial blood pressure by formation of alpha-methyl norepinephrine and by central stimulation of inhibitory alpha-adrenergic receptors

USUAL DOSAGE/ROUTE
ADULT
–PO: 250 mg 2–3 times daily initially, adjusting maintenance to a maximum of 3 gm/day
–IV: 250 mg–500 mg in 50–100 ml D_5W over 30–60 min every 6 hr not to exceed 1 gm every 6 hr

PEDIATRIC
–PO: 10 mg/kg/day in 2–4 divided doses initially, adjusting maintenance to a maximum of 65 mg/kg/day
–IV: 20–40 mg/kg/day in 4 divided doses, with a maximum of 65 mg/kg/day

ADVERSE/SIDE EFFECTS
RAPID
–NVD
–Dizziness
–Headache

GRADUAL
–Most common is drowsiness within 48–72 hr of therapy
–Hypotension and orthostatic hypotension
–General edema and weight gain due to salt and water retention

–Decreased urinary output
–Weakness
–Depression
–Psychosis
–Leukopenia
–Thrombocytopenia
–Hemolytic anemia
–Positive Coombs test
–Gynecomastia and lactation
–Impotence

CONTRAINDICATIONS

–Hypersensitivity
–Labile and mild hypertension
–Active hepatic disease or history of liver disease

SPECIAL PRECAUTIONS

–Pregnant or lactating patients
–Eclampsia
–Severe liver disease
–Cardiac disease

OTHER SPECIAL INFORMATION

–Onset of action is slow (6–12 hr PO, 4–6 hr IV).
–Full effect of drug is attained after 1–4 days of continued administration.
–This drug is often administered in conjunction with a thiazide diuretic such as HYDROCHLOROTHIAZIDE.
–Urine may darken.
–A positive direct Coombs test (laboratory test for antigen-antibody reactions and early diagnosis of hemolytic anemias) occurs in 10–20% of patients after 6–12 months and is dose related (rarely seen in daily doses less than 1 gm).
–Use with caution in patients on LEVODOPA; an additive hypotensive effect may occur.

ANTIDOTE

SEVERE REACTIONS

–D/C drug immediately and initiate appropriate treatment for symptoms.
–Treat low BP with a vasopressor such as DOPAMINE or METARAMINOL.

OTHER REACTIONS

–Notify physician of any side effects and initiate appropriate actions.

METHYLPREDNISOLONE, METHYLPREDNISOLONE ACETATE, METHYLPREDNISOLONE SODIUM SUCCINATE Depo-Medrol, Medrol, Solu-Medrol, and others

CLASS

–Corticosteroid (glucocorticoid)

USES

–Potent anti-inflammatory agent in management of ulcerative colitis, rheumatic fever, allergic and dermatologic disorders
–Shock
–Adrenal insufficiency
–Acute spinal cord injury

ACTION

–Synthetic adrenal steroid with similar glucocorticoid activity as HYDROCORTISONE, but considerably less sodium and water retention

USUAL DOSAGE/ROUTE

ADULT

–PO: 2–60 mg in 4 divided doses
–IM: 40–80 mg (ACETATE)

–IM or IV: 10–250 mg every 4 hr (SUCCINATE)
–*Shock:* IV: 100–250 mg at 2–6-hr intervals (SUCCINATE)
–Intraarticular: 4–30 mg (ACETATE)

PEDIATRIC

–PO: 0.117–1.66 mg/kg/day in 3–4 divided doses
–IM: 0.139–1.66 mg/kg/day in 1–2 divided doses
–IV: 117 meq/kg to 1.66 mg/kg in 3 or 4 divided doses (SUCCINATE)

ADVERSE/SIDE EFFECTS

RAPID

–Flushing
–Sweating
–Hypertension
–Tachycardia
–NVD

GRADUAL

–Euphoria
–Insomnia
–CHF
–Ecchymosis
–Edema
–Depression
–Thrombophlebitis
–Embolism
–Thrombocytopenia
–Osteoporosis
–Fractures
–Increased appetite
–Cataracts
–Glaucoma
–Peptic ulcer
–GI irritation or hemorrhage
–Hypokalemia
–Hyperglycemia
–Delayed wound healing
–Acne
–Muscle weakness
–Susceptibility to infection

CONTRAINDICATIONS
–Hypersensitivity
–Systemic fungal infections
–GI disease
–Renal disease
–Psychosis
–Hypertension
–Osteoporosis
–Cushing's syndrome
–Acute renal disease
–Emotional instability
–Children less than 2 years

SPECIAL PRECAUTIONS
–Pregnant or lactating patients
–Diabetes mellitus
–Glaucoma
–Osteoporosis
–Seizure disorders
–Myasthenia gravis
–CHF

OTHER SPECIAL INFORMATION
–Gradually reduce drug dosage to avoid adrenal crisis.
–Always titrate to lowest effective dose.
–Discard reconstituted solution after 48 hr.
–Give IM deep into gluteal muscle using 19G needle.
–Give PO with food or milk to decrease GI symptoms.
–Give IV dose slowly over one minute.
–Shock: give large IV doses over 3–15 minutes to prevent circulatory collapse.

ANTIDOTE

SEVERE REACTIONS
–D/C drug immediately and initiate appropriate treatment for symptoms.

OTHER REACTIONS
–Notify physician of any side effects and initiate appropriate actions.

METOCLOPRAMIDE HCL Clopra, Maxeran, Maxolon, Octamide, Reconomide, Reglan

CLASS

–Cholinergic (GI stimulant, antiemetic)

USES

–Management of esophageal reflux and gastric stasis (stimulates gastric emptying)
–Prevention of nausea and vomiting with chemotherapy, especially CISPLATIN
–Prevention of postoperative nausea and vomiting where nasogastric suctioning is undesirable
–To aid in small bowel intubation
–Used in combination with PROCHLORPERAZINE for migraine headache

ACTION

–Blocks dopamine receptors in chemoreceptor trigger zone of the CNS
–Stimulates motility of the upper GI tract and accelerates gastric emptying
–Enhances response to acetylcholine of tissue in the upper GI tract, which causes contraction of gastric muscle, relaxes pyloric and duodenal segments, increases peristalsis without stimulating secretions

USUAL DOSAGE/ROUTE

ADULT

–*Nausea and vomiting:* IM: 10–20 mg at end of procedure and every 4–6 hr as needed; IV: 2 mg/kg every 2 hr X 5 doses 30 min before administration of chemotherapy
–*Esophogeal reflux:* PO: 10–15 mg up to 4 times/day before meals and at bedtime (elderly patients may only need 5 mg doses because of increased sensitivity to therapeutic and adverse effects)
–*Diabetic gastric stasis* (The initial route is determined by the severity of symptoms): PO, IM: 10 mg 30 min before each

meal and at bedtime; IV: 10 mg administered slowly over a 1- to 2-min period

–*To facilitate small bowel intubation:* IV: 10 mg

PEDIATRIC

–IV (6–14 yr of age): 2.5 to 5.0 mg to facilitate small bowel intubation (do not exceed 0.5 mg/kg)

–IV (less than 6 yr of age): 0.1 mg/kg

ADVERSE/SIDE EFFECTS

RAPID

–Restlessness
–Drowsiness
–Fatigue
–Hypotension
–Supraventricular tachycardia
–Rash
–Irregular pulse

GRADUAL

–Extrapyramidal reactions (with large doses)
–Hepatotoxicity
–Gynecomastia
–Decreased libido
–Mental depression

CONTRAINDICATIONS

–Hypersensitivity to drug or PROCAINE or PROCAINAMIDE
–Pheochromocytoma
–History of seizure disorder
–GI obstruction, perforation, or hemorrhage
–Breast cancer

SPECIAL PRECAUTIONS

–History of hypertension
–Pregnant or lactating patients
–CHF
–Children and the elderly (increased incidence of extrapyramidal reactions)

OTHER SPECIAL INFORMATION

- This drug distributes widely into body tissues and fluids; crosses blood–brain barrier and placenta.
- Drug is metabolized by liver, excreted in urine; half-life of 4 hr.
- Teach patient and family to avoid driving or other hazardous activities until patient is stabilized on this medication.
- Teach patient to avoid alcohol or other CNS depressants that will enhance sedating properties of this drug.
- For IV doses greater than 10 mg, dilution should be done with 50 ml of a parenteral solution (NaCL, D_5W, LR) and infused over 15 min.

ANTIDOTE

SEVERE REACTIONS

- D/C drug immediately and initiate appropriate treatment for symptoms.

OTHER REACTIONS

- Notify physician of any side effects and initiate appropriate actions.

METOPROLOL TARTRATE Betaloc, Lopresor, Lopressor

CLASS

- Antihypertensive, beta-adrenergic blocker (antihypertensive, antianginal)

USES

- Mild-to-moderate hypertension
- Acute MI to reduce cardiovascular mortality
- Angina pectoris
- Treatment of mitral valve prolapse
- Prevention of vascular headaches

ACTION

–Blocks stimulation of beta-1 (myocardial) adrenergic receptors with less effect on beta-2 (pulmonary, vascular, or uterine) receptor sites to decrease the heart rate and BP

USUAL DOSAGE/ROUTE

ADULT

–*Hypertension, angina, myocardial infarction prophylaxis:* PO: 100–450 mg/day, single dose or twice a day
–*Myocardial infarction, acute:* initially IV: 5 mg every 2 min for 3 doses; then PO: 50 mg 15 min after last dose and every 6 hr for 48 hr; then maintenance dose of 100 mg twice daily for 3 months

PEDIATRIC

–Not for use in children

ADVERSE/SIDE EFFECTS

RAPID

–Bradycardia
–Peripheral vasoconstriction
–Hypotension
–N & V
–Dizziness
–Hiccups

GRADUAL

–Insomnia
–Fatigue
–Weakness
–Depression
–Impotence
–CHF
–AV block

CONTRAINDICATIONS

–Hypersensitivity to beta-blockers
–Uncompensated CHF
–Pulmonary edema
–Cardiogenic shock

–Bradycardia
–Heart block
–Sinus bradycardia
–Bronchial asthma

SPECIAL PRECAUTIONS

–Pregnant or lactating patients
–Children (safety not established)
–Diabetes mellitus
–Thyroid disease
–Liver disease
–Renal disease
–Major surgery
–Nonallergic bronchospasm

OTHER SPECIAL INFORMATION

–When given IV, keep patient recumbent for 3 hr.
–Monitor intake and output.
–Take apical/radial pulse before administering.
–Teach patient to take with, or immediately after, a meal.
–Avoid alcohol, smoking, and sodium intake while taking this drug.

ANTIDOTE

SEVERE REACTIONS

–D/C drug immediately and initiate appropriate treatment for symptoms.
–Treat overdose with gastric lavage, then ATROPINE IV for bradycardia; THEOPHYLLINE IV for bronchospasm; GLUCOSE IV for hypoglycemia; DIAZEPAM IV for seizures.
–Treat cardiac failure with a diuretic, DIGITALIS, OXYGEN, and hemodialysis.
–Treat hypotension with a vasopressor such as DOPAMINE.

OTHER REACTIONS

–Notify physician of any side effects and initiate appropriate actions.

MIDAZOLAM HCL Versed

CLASS

–General anesthetic (short-acting benzodiazepine), sedative hypnotic

USES

–Preoperative sedation and postoperative amnesia (induces sleepiness or drowsiness and relief of apprehension)
–Conscious sedation prior to short diagnostic procedures
–Induction of general anesthesia
–Intubation

ACTION

–Acts on many levels of the CNS to produce generalized CNS depression
–Effects may be mediated by gamma-aminobenzoic acid (GABA), an inhibitory neurotransmitter

USUAL DOSAGE/ROUTE

ADULT

–*Preoperative sedation/postoperative amnesia:* IM: 0.07–0.08 mg/kg (approx. 5 mg for an average adult) approx. 1 hr prior to surgery
–*Conscious sedation for short diagnostic procedures:* IV: 1–2.5 mg initially over 2 min; should be titrated slowly until desired effect is achieved (slurred speech). After another 2 min, more may be slowly administered. Rarely will more than 5 mg be needed. In the elderly (over 60 yr) or debilitated, initial dose should not exceed 1.5 mg, rarely needing doses greater than 3.5 mg.

PEDIATRIC

–Safety and effectiveness of Versed in children under 18 yr have not been established

ADVERSE/SIDE EFFECTS

RAPID

–Respiratory depression
–Excess sedation
–Laryngospasm
–Pain at IM site
–Phlebitis at IV site
–Cardiac arrest
–N & V
–Pruritis
–Hypotension

GRADUAL

–Blurred vision
–Toothache
–Insomnia
–Acid taste
–Headache

CONTRAINDICATIONS

–Hypersensitivity
–Acute narrow-angle glaucoma
–Acute alcohol intoxication
–Use in pregnancy (risk of congenital malformations)
–Shock or comatose patients
–Cross-sensitivity with other benzodiazapines

SPECIAL PRECAUTIONS

–Elderly and debilitated patients (dosage reduction required)
–Children (safety not established)
–Severe liver impairment
–Renal impairment
–CHF
–COPD

OTHER SPECIAL INFORMATION

–Prior to IV administration in any dose, there must be immediate availability of oxygen, resuscitative equipment, and skilled personnel for the maintenance of a patent airway.

–Monitor patients continuously for signs of underventilation or apnea.
–Monitor vital signs during the recovery period.

ANTIDOTE

SEVERE REACTIONS

–D/C drug immediately and initiate appropriate treatment for symptoms.
–For hypotension, give a vasopressor such as NOREPINEPHRINE.
–For cardiac/respiratory arrest, implement ALS procedures as appropriate.
–For overdose, give the cholinergic PHYSOSTIGMINE to reverse CNS effects.

OTHER REACTIONS

–Notify physician of any side effects and initiate appropriate actions.

MORPHINE SULFATE Astramorph, Duramorph, Morphine, MS, MS Contin, and others

CLASS

–Narcotic analgesic (opiate)

USES

–Severe pain when non-narcotic analgesics have failed
–Sedation and hypnosis in presence of pain, particularly of myocardial infarction
–Preanesthetic medication
–Dyspnea associated with acute left ventricular failure and pulmonary edema

ACTION

–Depressed pain impulse transmission by acting on opiate receptors (concentrated in the limbic system, central part of the thalamus, and parts of the spinal cord and intestine), inhibiting ascending pain pathways

USUAL DOSAGE/ROUTE

ADULT

–PO: 10–30 mg every 4 hr or 30 mg every 8–12 hr for extended release preparations
–Rectal: 10–30 mg every 4 hr
–Epidural: 2–10 mg/day or 0.6–0.8 mg/kg/day continuous infusion
–Intrathecal: 0.2–1.0 mg single dose
–SC, IM: 5–20 mg every 4 hr as needed
–IV: 2.5–15 mg in 4–5 ml sterile water for injection; inject slowly over a 4–5-min period every 4 hr as needed
–IV infusion: 15 mg loading dose, then 0.8–10.0 mg/hr titrated for pain relief

PEDIATRIC

–SC: 0.1–0.2 mg/kg every 4 hr not to exceed 15 mg per dose
–IM, IV: 50–100 mcg/kg not to exceed 10 mg per dose

ADVERSE/SIDE EFFECTS

RAPID

–Respiratory depression
–Dizziness
–Sedation
–Euphoria
–Paradoxical CNS stimulation (restlessness, tremor, delirium)
–Headache
–Sweating
–N & V
–Hypotension
–Syncope
–Anaphylaxis
–Urticaria, pruritus
–Constricted pupils
–Pain, phlebitis at injection site
–Depressed cough reflex

–Bradycardia
–Palpitations

CONTRAINDICATIONS

–Hypersensitivity
–Pregnancy or lactation
–Increased intracranial pressure
–Convulsive disorders
–Respiratory diseases, particularly asthma
–Undiagnosed acute abdominal conditions

SPECIAL PRECAUTIONS

–Hypothyroidism
–Head trauma
–Adrenal insufficiency
–Alcoholism
–Elderly
–Debilitated patients
–Prostatic hypertrophy
–Addictive personality
–Renal disease
–Liver disease
–Reduced blood volume
–Hypotension
–Compromised or slowed respiratory rate

OTHER SPECIAL INFORMATION

–Parenteral administration produces greater reliability in absorption rate with onset of action within 20 min, peak ½–1½ hr, and duration up to 7 hr.
–Approximately 90% of dose is excreted, primarily in the urine, within 24 hr.
–Continued use may produce drug dependence.
–Use with caution and in reduced dosage in patients receiving other CNS depressants, including alcohol.
–Safe use is not established in pregnancy; crosses the placental barrier and may cause fetal respiratory depression.
–Depth and rate of respirations are diminished by this drug; watch for clinical signs of hypoxia as well as decreased rate.

ANTIDOTE

SEVERE REACTIONS

–D/C drug immediately and initiate appropriate treatment for symptoms.

–Treat overdose with NALOXONE 0.2–0.8 mg IV repeated as necessary or as a continuous infusion, OXYGEN, IV fluids.

–Treat hypotension with vasopressors such as DOPAMINE or METARAMINOL or NOREPINEPHRINE.

OTHER REACTIONS

–Notify physician of any side effects and initiate appropriate actions.

NADOLOL Corgard

CLASS
–Beta-adrenergic blocker (antihypertensive, antianginal)

USES
–Chronic stable angina
–Mild-to-moderate hypertension
–Tachydysrhythmias
–Migraine prophylaxis
–Thyrotoxicosis

ACTION
–Blocks stimulation of beta-1 (myocardial) and beta-2 (pulmonary) receptor sites to lower heart rate and BP

USUAL DOSAGE/ROUTE
ADULT
–PO: 40 mg once per day, increasing by 40–80 mg every 3–7 days until acquired effects achieved, up to 320 mg/day
–*Angina*, maintenance: 40–240 mg/day
–*Hypertension*, maintenance: 40–320 mg/day

PEDIATRIC
–Safe use in children not established

ADVERSE/SIDE EFFECTS
RAPID
–Palpitations
–AV block
–Laryngospasm
–Bronchospasm
–Dyspnea/wheezing
–Chest pain
–Flushing
–Conduction disturbances
–NVD

–Rash
–Dizziness

GRADUAL
–Hypotension
–Bradycardia
–Pharyngitis
–Agranulocytosis
–Thrombocytopenia
–Hepatomegaly
–Flatulence
–Pancreatitis
–Taste distortion
–Depression
–Fever
–Raynaud's phenomenon
–Fatigue/weakness

CONTRAINDICATIONS
–Hypersensitivity
–CHF/PE
–Cardiogenic shock
–2nd- or 3rd-degree heart block
–Bronchospastic disease
–Bradycardia
–Hypotension
–COPD
–Asthma

SPECIAL PRECAUTIONS
–Pregnant or lactating patients
–Diabetes mellitus (masks hypoglycemia)
–Renal disease (requires reduced dosage)
–Hyperthyroidism
–Peripheral vascular disease
–Myasthenia gravis
–Children

OTHER SPECIAL INFORMATION
–This drug is long acting; half-life = 16–20 hr; duration = 17–24 hr.

–Assess BP, pulse, respirations prior to therapy and periodically during therapy for decreases.
–Perform daily weights (drug may cause fluid retention).
–Administer PO drug with at least 8 ounces of water.
–Headache, light-headedness, decreased BP may indicate a need to decrease the dosage.
–Do not discontinue abruptly.
–This drug may lower blood glucose and mask signs of hypoglycemia in diabetic patients.

ANTIDOTE

SEVERE REACTIONS
–D/C drug immediately and initiate appropriate treatment for symptoms.
–Treat bradycardia with IV ATROPINE SULFATE.
–Treat hypotension with an IV vasopressor such as DOPAMINE or METARAMINOL.
–Treat bronchospasm with IV THEOPHYLLINE.
–Treat dysrhythmias with an IV cardiac glycoside such as DIGOXIN.

OTHER REACTIONS
–Notify physician of any side effects and initiate appropriate actions.

NALBUPHINE HCL Nubain

CLASS
–Non-narcotic analgesic (opiate)

USES
–Moderate-to-severe pain
–Preoperative analgesia
–Obstetrical analgesia during labor

ACTION

–Depresses pain impulse transmission by acting on opiate receptors at the spinal cord level, inhibiting ascending pain pathways

USUAL DOSAGE/ROUTE

ADULT

–SC, IM, IV: 10–20 mg every 3–6 hr as needed, not to exceed 160 mg/day

PEDIATRIC

–Safe use in children not established

ADVERSE/SIDE EFFECTS

RAPID

–Sedation
–Euphoria
–Dizziness
–Headache
–Sweaty/clammy skin
–N & V
–Rash
–Dry mouth
–Diaphoresis
–Respiratory depression
–Hypotension
–Bradycardia
–Palpitations
–Urinary urgency

GRADUAL

–Anorexia
–Constipation
–Cramps

CONTRAINDICATIONS

–Hypersensitivity
–Increased intracranial pressure
–Narcotic addiction
–Impaired respiratory disease, particularly bronchial asthma

–Children under 18 years
–Impaired renal or hepatic function
–Impaired liver function
–Undiagnosed abdominal pain

SPECIAL PRECAUTIONS

–Head trauma
–Hypothyroidism
–Adrenal insufficiency
–Alcoholism
–Elderly
–Debilitated patients
–Prostatic hypertrophy
–Pregnancy or lactating patients
–Addictive personality
–Severe heart disease

OTHER SPECIAL INFORMATION

–Use with extreme caution as preoperative analgesic for biliary tract surgery; causes spasm of the sphincter of Oddi.
–Low abuse potential, though withdrawal after long-term use may produce symptoms of drug dependence.
–Reduce dosage if used in combination with other CNS depressants.
–Use with extreme caution in patients with nausea or vomiting associated with myocardial infarction.
–Onset = 2–3 min after IV administration, less than 15 min after SC or IM injection; plasma half-life = 5 hr; duration = 3–6 hr.

ANTIDOTE

SEVERE REACTIONS

–D/C drug immediately and initiate appropriate treatment for symptoms.
–Treat overdose with NALOXONE 0.2–0.8 mg IV repeated as necessary, or as a continuous infusion, OXYGEN, IV fluids.
–Treat hypotension with vasopressors such as DOPAMINE, METARAMINOL, or NOREPINEPHRINE.

OTHER REACTIONS

–Notify physician of any side effects and initiate appropriate actions.

NALOXONE HCL Narcan

CLASS

–Narcotic antagonist

USES

–Complete or partial reversal of narcotic depression, including respiratory and CNS depression induced by natural and synthetic narcotics, PROPOXYPHENE (Darvocet-N), and PENTAZOCINE (Talwin)

–Diagnosis of suspected opiate overdosage

–Experimental usage in septic shock to improve cardiovascular function

ACTION

–Pure narcotic antagonist action, competing with opioid agonists for binding sites on nerve cells

USUAL DOSAGE/ROUTE

ADULT

–*Narcotic overdose:* SC, IM, IV: 1–2 mg repeated at 2–3-minute intervals times 2–3 doses as needed

–*Postoperative respiratory depression:* IV: 0.1–0.2 mg repeated at 2–3-minute intervals titrated to desired degree of reversal

PEDIATRIC

–SC, IM, IV: 0.01 mg/kg, repeated at 2–3-minute intervals times 2–3 doses as needed

–*Neonatal respiratory depression:* IV: 0.01 mg/kg into umbilical vein, and may repeat at 2–3-minute intervals times 2–3 doses as needed

ADVERSE/SIDE EFFECTS

RAPID

EXCESSIVE DOSAGE
–Reversal of analgesia
–Increased blood pressure
–Hyperventilation
–Slight drowsiness
–Tremor
–Elevated partial thromboplastin time (PTT)

TOO RAPID REVERSAL
–N & V
–Ventricular fibrillation
–Sweating
–Tachycardia

GRADUAL
–None reported

CONTRAINDICATIONS
–Hypersensitivity
–Respiratory depression caused by non-narcotic analgesics
–Known or suspected narcotic addiction
–Cardiac irritability

SPECIAL PRECAUTIONS
–Pregnant or lactating patients
–Narcotic-dependent patients
–Cardiovascular disease
–Neonates of narcotic-dependent mothers

OTHER SPECIAL INFORMATION
–IV route is preferred.
–Monitor surgical and obstetrical patients for bleeding secondary to elevated PTT.
–Does not produce respiratory depression, psychotomimetic effects, or pupillary constriction
–Onset of action: IV = 2 min; SC, IM = 2–5 min; duration of action = 3–5 hr depending on dosage and route of administration; plasma half-life = 64 min.

–This drug is metabolized in the liver and excreted in urine.
–Repeated dosage may be necessary depending on the narcotic being antagonized.

ANTIDOTE

SEVERE REACTIONS

–D/C drug immediately and initiate appropriate treatment for symptoms.

OTHER REACTIONS

–Notify physician of any side effects and initiate appropriate actions.

NAPROXEN, NAPROXEN SODIUM
Anaprox, Naprosyn

CLASS

–Nonsteriodal (anti-inflammatory agent)

USES

–Rheumatoid arthritis, osteoarthritis, juvenile arthritis
–Ankylosing spondylitis
–Tendonitis and bursitis
–Acute gout
–To relieve mild-to-moderate pain
–Treatment of primary dysmenorrhea

ACTION

–Inhibits prostaglandin synthesis by decreasing an enzyme needed for biosynthesis
–Possesses analgesic, anti-inflammatory, and antipyretic properties

USUAL DOSAGE/ROUTE

ADULT

–*Treatment of rheumatoid arthritis, osteoarthritis, and ankylosing spondylitis, gout:* PO, tablet, or suspension: 250

mg, 375 mg, or 500 mg 2 times/day up to 1500 mg per day when a higher level of analgesic/anti-inflammatory activity is required

–*For mild-to-moderate pain, primary dysmenorrhea, and acute tendonitis and bursitis:* PO, tablet or suspension: Initial dose of 500 mg followed by 250 mg every 6–8 hr as required, not to exceed 1,250 mg

PEDIATRIC

–*For juvenile arthritis:* suspension: 10 mg/kg given in 2 divided doses

ADVERSE/SIDE EFFECTS

RAPID

–N & V
–Drowsiness
–Dizziness
–Rash
–Heartburn
–Tachycardia
–Thirst

GRADUAL

–Constipation
–Abdominal pain
–Jaundice
–Cholestatic hepatitis
–Dry mouth
–Peptic ulcer
–Confusion
–Anxiety
–Depression
–Nephrotoxicity
–Tinnitus
–Blurred vision
–Photosensitivity

CONTRAINDICATIONS

–Hypersensitivity to drug or ASPIRIN
–Severe renal disease
–Severe liver disease

–Ulcer disease
–Active GI bleed
–Asthma

SPECIAL PRECAUTIONS

–Pregnant or lactating patients
–Severe cardiovascular disease
–Children
–Elderly
–Bleeding disorders

OTHER SPECIAL INFORMATION

–275 mg NAPROXEN SODIUM = 250 mg NAPROXEN.
–BUN, serum creatinine, CBC, and liver function tests should be evaluated periodically in patients receiving prolonged courses of therapy.
–Assess audiometric and ophthalmic exams before, during, and after treatment.
–Administer with food to decrease GI symptoms; best to take on empty stomach to facilitate absorption.
–Teach patient/family to report blurred vision and roaring in ears (may indicate toxicity).
–Therapeutic effects may take up to one month.
–Drug reduces the antihypertensive effect of PROPANOLOL and other beta-blockers.

ANTIDOTE

SEVERE REACTIONS

–D/C drug immediately and initiate appropriate treatment for symptoms.

OTHER REACTIONS

–Notify physician of any side effects and initiate appropriate actions.

NIFEDIPINE Adalat, Procardia

CLASS
–Calcium channel blocker (antagonist), antianginal, coronary vasodilator

USES
–Supraventricular tachydysrhythmia
–Angina pectoris
–Hypertension (sustained release only)

ACTION
–Inhibits the transmembrane influx of calcium ions into cardiac muscle causing coronary vasodilation and lowered blood pressure

USUAL DOSAGE/ROUTE
ADULT
–PO: 10–30 mg 3 or 4 times a day not to exceed 180 mg/day
–SL: 10 mg repeated in 20–30 minutes

PEDIATRIC
–Safe use in children not established

ADVERSE/SIDE EFFECTS
RAPID
–Dizziness
–Light-headedness
–Flushing
–Heat sensation
–Headache
–Weakness
–Nervousness
–Nausea
–Dyspnea
–Cough
–Wheezing

–Hypotension
–Syncope
–Tachycardia

GRADUAL
–Sore throat
–Nasal congestion
–Abdominal discomfort
–Hepatitis
–Flatulence
–Muscle cramps
–CHF
–Ankle edema

CONTRAINDICATIONS
–Sick sinus syndrome
–Hypersensitivity to drug
–Hypotension

SPECIAL PRECAUTIONS
–Severe hepatic disease
–CHF
–Aortic stenosis
–Pregnant or lactating patients
–Children

OTHER SPECIAL INFORMATION
–Careful monitoring of blood pressure during the initial administration and titration is suggested.
–Sublingual NITROGLYCERIN may be taken as required for the control of acute angina during titration of this drug.
–Doses as high as 320 mg/day have been used in clinical trials.

ANTIDOTE
SEVERE REACTIONS
–D/C drug immediately and initiate appropriate treatment for symptoms.
–Treat overdose with defibrilation.
–Treat AV block with ATROPINE SULFATE.

–Treat hypotension with vasopressors such as DOPAMINE, METARAMINOL, NOREPINEPHRINE.

OTHER REACTIONS

–Notify physician of any side effects and initiate appropriate actions.

NIMODIPINE Nimotop

CLASS

–Calcium channel blocker (cerebral vasodilator)

USES

–Prevention of cerebral vasospasm in early management of subarachnoid hemorrhage

ACTION

–Vasodilation by slowing calcium channels in vascular smooth muscle, and also decreases neurological impairment by prevention of cerebral arterial spasm

USUAL DOSAGE/ROUTE

ADULT

–PO: 60 mg every 4 hr for 21 days (should be started within 96 hr of subarachnoid hemorrhage)

PEDIATRIC

–Safe use in children not established

ADVERSE/SIDE EFFECTS

RAPID

–Hypotension
–Bradycardia
–Shortness of breath
–Confusion
–Wheezing
–Rash

GRADUAL
–Psychiatric disturbances
–Headache
–Dizziness
–Bradycardia
–Peripheral edema
–Nausea
–Constipation
–Muscle cramps

CONTRAINDICATIONS
–Hypersensitivity
–Pregnant or lactating patients
–Second- or third-degree heart block
–Hypotension
–Renal failure
–Children

SPECIAL PRECAUTIONS
–Severe hypertension
–Liver disease
–Elderly

OTHER SPECIAL INFORMATION
–This drug increases hypotension if used with antihypertensives, alcohol, or nitrates.
–There is increased risk of toxicity if used with CIMETIDINE.
–If patient unable to swallow capsules or has NG tube, poke a hole in ends of capsule with 18G needle and extract contents with syringe.
–A dosage reduction of ½ is required in patients with liver impairment, because the drug is extensively metabolized in the liver.

ANTIDOTE
SEVERE REACTIONS
–D/C drug immediately and initiate appropriate treatment for symptoms.
–Treat bradycardia with sympathomimetics or ATROPINE.

–Treat hypotension with vasopressors such as DOPAMINE.
–Treat cardiac failure with cardiac pacing.
–Treat calcium channel blocker overdose with IV CALCIUM GLUCONATE.

OTHER REACTIONS

–Notify physician of any side effects and initiate appropriate actions.

NITROGLYCERIN, (GLYCERYL TRINITRATE)
Cardabid, Carobid, Nitro-Bid, Nitrocap, Nitrocels, Nitrodisc, Nitro-Dur, Nitrol, Nitrol Ointment, Nitrol Paste, Nitrostat, Nitrostat IV, Tridil, and others

CLASS

–Cardiac vasodilator, antianginal

USES

–For the treatment and prevention of acute anginal attacks
–Sublingual tablets used to treat acute anginal episode as well as prior to event that may evoke angina
–Ointment used for prevention of attacks, particularly nocturnal anginal attacks
–CHF associated with acute MI
–Pulmonary edema

ACTION

–Direct relaxation of vascular smooth muscle producing vasodilation accompanied by decreased systemic vascular resistance, decreased blood pressure, and decreased cardiac output secondary to reduced venous return to heart (decreased preload and afterload)
–Reduces myocardial oxygen consumption to provide relief of anginal attacks

USUAL DOSAGE/ROUTE

ADULT

–SL: Dissolve 1 tablet (0.15–0.6 mg) under tongue, repeat every 5 min as needed until relief obtained up to 3 tablets

–Topical: 1–2 inches (2% ointment) as squeezed from tube every 3–4 hours as necessary; some patients may require up to 4–5 inches. Optimal dose determined by starting with ½ inch and increasing for each successive application until headache occurs, then decrease to largest dose that does not cause headache; may be applied anywhere on skin that is free of hair.

–IV: 5 mcg/min, then increase by 5 mcg/min every 3–5 min until desired response

PEDIATRIC

–Not for use in children

ADVERSE/SIDE EFFECTS

RAPID

–Tachycardia
–Syncope
–Weakness
–Flushing
–Skin rash
–Postural hypotension
–N & V
–Involuntary passage of urine and feces
–Palpitation
–Hypotension

GRADUAL

–Transient headache
–Dry mouth
–Blurred vision
–Dizziness
–Vertigo
–Exfoliative dermatitis

CONTRAINDICATIONS

–Hypersensitivity to nitrates/nitrites
–Severe anemia

–Hypotension
–Increased intracranial pressure
–Head trauma
–Cerebral hemorrhage
–Glaucoma

SPECIAL PRECAUTIONS

–Patients on antihypertensives
–Pregnant or lactating patients

OTHER SPECIAL INFORMATION

–0.15 mg = 1/400 gr; 0.3 mg = 1/200 gr; 0.4 mg = 1/150 gr; 0.6 mg = 1/100 gr.
–Sublingual tablet should be placed under tongue or in buccal pouch and allowed to dissolve naturally; do not swallow until entirely dissolved.
–Potent sublingual NITROGLYCERIN will cause a burning or tingling sensation under the tongue.
–Persons should sit or lie down before taking sublingual NITROGLYCERIN; hypotensive effect is greater in the upright position.
–With IV forms of this drug, be sure to use special nonabsorbing IV tubing supplied by the manufacturer and use a glass bottle and controlled infusion pump (up to 80% may be absorbed into plastic).
–Onset of action of sublingual tablet is 1–3 min, duration up to 30 min; topical ointment acts in 30–60 min, duration 3–7 hr; IV acts immediately, duration is variable.
–After squeezing ointment from tube, use applicator paper to spread thin layer on skin; do not rub or massage; wear gloves on hands during application and wash hands afterwards.
–Store NITROGLYCERIN tablets in original container, tightly closed in a cool, dry place; discard unused portion 3 months after original container is opened.
–Discontinue drug if blurred vision or dry mouth occur.
–Because of possibility of tolerance developing with prolonged use, smallest effective dose should be used.
–Rotate ointment application sites to prevent dermal inflam-

mation and sensitization; remove ointment from previous site before reapplication.
–Treatment should be terminated by gradually decreasing the dosage and frequency of applications.

ANTIDOTE

SEVERE REACTIONS
–D/C drug immediately and initiate appropriate treatment for symptoms.
–Treat hypotension with a vasopressor such as DOPAMINE.

OTHER REACTIONS
–Notify physician of any side effects and initiate appropriate actions.

NITROGLYCERIN LINGUAL SPRAY
Nitrolingual Spray

CLASS
–Nitrate vasodilator (antianginal, coronary vasodilator)

USES
–Acute relief of an attack of angina pectoris
–Prophylaxis of angina pectoris due to coronary artery disease

ACTION
–Increases coronary blood flow by dilating coronary arteries and improving collateral flow to ischemic regions
–Produces vasodilation (venous greater than arterial) promoting peripheral pooling of blood, decreasing venous return to the heart
–Decreases left ventricular, end-diastolic pressure and left ventricular end-diastolic volume (preload)
–Reduces myocardial oxygen consumption

USUAL DOSAGE/ROUTE

ADULT

–0.4 mg/spray: 1–2 sprays, may be repeated every 3–5 min for a total of 3 sprays (should spray onto or under the tongue); the spray should not be inhaled.

PEDIATRIC

–Not for use in children

ADVERSE/SIDE EFFECTS

RAPID

–Headache
–Hypotension, orthostatic hypotension
–Cutaneous vasodilation
–Flushing
–Tachycardia
–Dizziness

GRADUAL

–Apprehension
–Weakness
–N & V
–Pallor

CONTRAINDICATIONS

–Known hypersensitivity or idiosyncrasy to drug or other nitrates or nitrites
–Pericardial tamponade
–Severe anemia
–Constrictive pericarditis

SPECIAL PRECAUTIONS

–Severe hypotension
–Head trauma
–Cerebral hemorrhage
–Pregnant or lactating patients
–Glaucoma

OTHER SPECIAL INFORMATION

–Monitor blood pressure and pulse prior to and following administration.

–Caution patient to make position changes slowly to minimize orthostatic hypotension.
–Instruct patient to lift tongue and spray dose under tongue.
–Physical dependence also occurs; chest pain, acute myocardial infarction, and even sudden death have occurred during temporary withdrawal of nitroglycerin from workers (industrial workers exposed to nitroglycerin).

ANTIDOTE

SEVERE REACTIONS

–D/C drug immediately and initiate appropriate treatment for symptoms.
–For hypotension give a vasopressor such as NOREPINEPHRINE.

OTHER REACTIONS

–Notify physician of any side effects and initiate appropriate actions.

NITROPRUSSIDE SODIUM Nipride, Nitropress

CLASS

–Antihypertensive

USES

–Hypertensive crises, for short-term, rapid reduction of blood pressure
–To produce controlled hypotension during surgery to reduce bleeding

ACTION

–Similar action as nitrates; acts directly on vascular smooth muscle producing peripheral vasodilation leading to significant decrease in arterial blood pressure

USUAL DOSAGE/ROUTE

ADULT (IV use only)

- 50 mg diluted in 2–3 ml of D_5W and added to 250–1000 ml of D_5W to run at 0.5–8.0 mcg/kg/min
- Infusion rate greater than 10 mcg/kg/min should be immediately stopped if adequate reduction in blood pressure not obtained in 10 min

PEDIATRIC

- Not for use in children

ADVERSE/SIDE EFFECTS

RAPID (too fast reduction in blood pressure)

- Nausea
- Abdominal pain
- Nasal stuffiness
- Diaphoresis
- Headache
- Dizziness
- Apprehension
- Restlessness
- Muscle twitching
- Retrosternal discomfort
- Palpitations
- Increase or transient decrease in pulse

RAPID (overdose)

- Profound hypotension
- Tinnitus
- Blurred vision
- Fatigue
- Metabolic acidosis
- Pink skin color
- Areflexia
- Unconsciousness
- Faint heart sounds

GRADUAL

- None reported

CONTRAINDICATIONS

–Hypersensitivity
–Treatment of compensatory hypertension (AV shunt, coarctation of aorta)
–Decreased cerebral perfusion
–Pregnancy
–Children
–Hypothyroidism
–Hyponatremia

SPECIAL PRECAUTIONS

–Pregnant or lactating patients
–Renal disease
–Liver disease
–Elderly
–Vitamin B_{12} deficiency

OTHER SPECIAL INFORMATION

–Prepared solution must be immediately wrapped in foil to protect from light.
–Solution must be discarded after 4 hr.
–Discard if solution is highly colored; normally it has a light brown tint.
–This drug must be administered with infusion pump.
–Blood pressure must be monitored every 5–15 min; arterial pressure line is recommended.
–Onset of action = 1–2 min; duration = 1–10 min after infusion is terminated.
–Plasma cyanide levels and thiocyanate levels should be measured within 1–2 days after therapy initiated and measured periodically if therapy prolonged.
–This drug is not compatible with other medication, IV fluids.
–Effect is potentiated by concurrent use of other antihypertensive agents.

ANTIDOTE

SEVERE REACTIONS

–D/C drug immediately and initiate appropriate treatment for symptoms.

–Treat overdose with AMYL NITRATE inhalation for 15–30 sec every minute until IV SODIUM NITRATE infusion begun at 2.5–5.0 ml/min. up to 10–15 ml, then administer SODIUM THIOSULFATE 12.5 gm in 50 ml D_5W IV over 10 min and may repeat at 1/2 dose if necessary.
–Treat hypotension with vasopressors such as DOPAMINE, METARAMINOL, or NOREPINEPHRINE.

OTHER REACTIONS

–Notify physician of any side effects and initiate appropriate actions.

NITROUS OXIDE GAS Nitrous Oxide Gas

CLASS

–Inhalation anesthetic/analgesic

USES

–Produces weak anesthesia as a single agent in brief procedures or in combination with other anesthetics to produce long-term anesthesia

ACTION

–Acts at level of CNS to produce mild anesthesia and powerful analgesia; does not cause skeletal muscle relaxation

USUAL DOSAGE/ROUTE

ADULT AND PEDIATRIC

–Always administered with minimum of 28% oxygen
–Titrated according to desired analgesia/anesthesia
–Semiclosed induction via anesthetic machine using masks or endotracheal tube

ADVERSE/SIDE EFFECTS

RAPID

–Hypoxia
–N & V (minimal)

–Delirium
–Respiratory depression
–Dysrhythmias
–Vasodilation producing hypotension, hypothermia, tachypnea, tachycardia

GRADUAL

–Expansion of air pockets in abdomen, chest, and skull
–Sodium retention
–Decreased urine output (temporary)

CONTRAINDICATIONS

–Hypersensitivity
–Myocardial damage
–Cardiovascular collapse
–Preexisting uncorrected hypoxia
–Uncontrolled dysrhythmias
–Head injury
–COPD
–Hepatic failure

SPECIAL PRECAUTIONS

–Patients susceptible to hyperpyrexia (abnormal activity; restlessness)
–Ventricular dysrhythmias

OTHER SPECIAL INFORMATION

–This drug is a nonexplosive anesthetic gas.
–Vital signs must be continuously monitored during and after administration until patient is stable.
–Drug is primarily excreted through the lungs and is partially excreted by the liver.
–Strict I & O for signs/symptoms of circulatory overload after administration is required due to the possible stimulation of ADH secretion.

ANTIDOTE

SEVERE REACTIONS

–D/C drug immediately and initiate appropriate treatment for symptoms.

OTHER REACTIONS

–Notify physician of any side effects and initiate appropriate actions.

NOREPINEPHRINE, LEVARTERENOL BITARTRATE   Levarterenol, Levophed

CLASS

–Adrenergic, vasopressor

USES

–Maintenance of blood pressure in acute hypotension
–Central vasomotor depression
–Myocardial infarction

ACTION

–Powerful vasoconstriction (alpha-adrenergic), potent inotropic stimulator of heart, and dilator of coronary arteries (beta-adrenergic)
–Increases blood pressure, coronary patency blood flow, and cardiac output

USUAL DOSAGE/ROUTE

ADULT

–IV only: 2–8 ml of a 0.2% solution added to 500 ml of D_5W for continuous infusion and titrated by BP changes; average infusion rate is 8–12 mcg/min initially, then 2–4 mcg/min maintenance titrated by BP changes

PEDIATRIC

–IV only: 1 ml of a 0.2% solution added to 250 ml of D_5W for continuous infusion and titrated by BP changes; average infusion rate is 1–2 mcg/min titrated by BP changes

ADVERSE/SIDE EFFECTS

RAPID

–Hypertension
–Headache

–Increased peripheral resistance (vasoconstriction)
–Palpitations
–Tachycardia
–Ectopic beats
–Angina

GRADUAL
–N & V
–Tissue sloughing & gangrene with extravasation

CONTRAINDICATIONS
–Hypersensitivity to the drug
–Hypotension from blood loss
–Tachydysrhythmias
–Pregnancy
–Persons receiving cyclopropane and halothane anesthesia
–Pheochromocytoma

SPECIAL PRECAUTIONS
–Lactating patients
–Embolism
–Elderly
–Peripheral vascular disease
–Hypertension
–Hyperthyroidism

OTHER SPECIAL INFORMATION
–Drug is only given per continuous IV drip.
–Establish baseline blood pressure and continue to monitor blood pressure and pulse every 2–5 min during drug administration.
–Infiltration of drug will cause tissue sloughing; use extravasation procedure.
–Use a large vein for drug administration to decrease the risk of poor limb circulation.

ANTIDOTE

SEVERE REACTIONS
–D/C drug immediately and initiate appropriate treatment for symptoms.

–Treat bradycardia with ATROPINE.
–Treat overdose with fluids and electrolyte replacement.

OTHER REACTIONS

–Notify physician of any side effects and initiate appropriate actions.

OXYCODONE HCL Oxycet, Percocet, Percodan, Roxicet, Tylox

CLASS
–Narcotic analgesic

USES
–Relieve moderate-to-moderately severe pain that may occur with neuralgia, bursitis, dislocations, simple fractures, and similar injuries
–Relieve postoperative, postextractional, and postpartum pain

ACTION
–Acts similarly to MORPHINE to bind with the opiate receptor in the CNS to produce mild sedation, analgesia, and euphoria

USUAL DOSAGE/ROUTE

ADULT
–PO: 5 mg every 3–6 hr as needed, or 10 mg 3–4 times a day as needed

PEDIATRIC
–(6–12 yr) PO: 1.25 mg every 6 hr as needed
–(> 12 yr) PO: 2.5 mg every 6 hr as needed

ADVERSE/SIDE EFFECTS

RAPID
–Light-headedness
–Dizziness
–Sedation (mild)
–N & V
–Dysphoria
–Euphoria
–Pruritis
–Orthostatic hypotension
–Respiratory depression

GRADUAL
- Constipation
- Urinary retention
- Physical dependence
- Psychological dependence

CONTRAINDICATIONS
- Hypersensitivity to the drug or any of the ingredients
- CNS trauma
- Increased intracranial pressure
- Hepatic dysfunction
- Renal dysfunction
- Pregnancy or lactation
- Severe respiratory disease
- Known drug dependence

SPECIAL PRECAUTIONS
- Hypothyroidism
- Adrenal insufficiency
- Alcoholism
- Elderly
- Debilitated patients
- Prostatic hypertrophy

OTHER SPECIAL INFORMATION
- Onset of action = 10–15 min; peak = 30–60 min; duration = 3–6 hr.
- Detoxification occurs in the liver and kidneys with excretion primarily in urine.
- Avoid concurrent use with other CNS depressants.
- This drug should be taken with milk or after meals.
- Caution patient against driving a car or operating hazardous equipment while consuming drug.
- Watch for ACETAMINOPHEN hepatic toxicity with excessive doses or overdoses of this drug.
- Percodan contains 4.5 mg OXYCODONE HCL, 0.38 mg OXYCODONE TEREPHTHALATE, 224 mg ASPIRIN, 160 mg PHENACETIN, and 32 mg CAFFEINE.
- Percocet contains 5 mg OXYCODONE HCL and 325 mg ACETAMINOPHEN.

ANTIDOTE

SEVERE REACTIONS

–D/C drug immediately and initiate appropriate treatment for symptoms.

–Treat overdose with NALOXONE 0.2–0.8 mg IV, OXYGEN, IV fluids.

–Treat hypotension with vasopressors such as DOPAMINE, METARAMINOL, or NOREPINEPHRINE.

OTHER REACTIONS

–Notify physician of any side effects and initiate appropriate actions.

OXYGEN GAS Oxygen, O_2

CLASS

–Gas

USES

–Prevent and treat hypoxemia to reduce tissue damage and reduce energy expenditure

–In conjunction with anesthesia or Nitrous Oxide Gas administration

–Maintain functional readiness of transplant tissues

–Ischemic chest pain

–Oxygenate blood during coronary bypass surgery

–Increase healing and decrease scarring in burns

ACTION

–Elevates arterial oxygen tension and increases hemoglobin–oxygen saturation to improve tissue oxygenation necessary to prevent cellular damage and death

USUAL DOSAGE/ROUTE

ADULT AND PEDIATRIC

–Dependent on degree of hypoxia and underlying cause

WITH SPONTANEOUS RESPIRATIONS

–Nasal cannula: 1–6 liters/min, delivers 22–40%
–Nasal catheter: 1–6 liters/min, delivers 22–40%
–Standard face mask: 6–12 liters/min, delivers 22–40%
–Reservoir mask: 6–10 liters/min, delivers 50–99%
–Venturi mask, used for chronic obstructive lung disease: 4–10 liters/min, delivers 24%, 28%, 35%, and 40%
–Face tent: 5–8 liters/min

RESPIRATORY DEPRESSION-ARREST

–Mouth-to-mouth rescue breathing: 16–17%
–Bag-valve-mask: 15 liters/min, delivers 40–90%
–Endotracheal tube, esophageal obturator airway, or tracheostomy tube with manually triggered, oxygen-powered resuscitator: up to 100 liters/min, delivers up to 100%
–Volume mechanical ventilation: 21–100 liters/min, delivers 21–100%

ADVERSE/SIDE EFFECTS

RAPID

–None reported

GRADUAL

–Drying of mucous membranes, thickening of secretions, reduced ciliary function
–Pulmonary irritation characterized by coughing, dyspnea, and substernal pain with prolonged administration at high concentrations
–Oxygen toxicity characterized by increased alveolar dead space, shunting, and decreased vital capacity
–Grand mal seizures with administration greater than 2½ atmospheres
–Retrolental fibroplasia and subsequent permanent blindness in premature infants with administration at arterial oxygen tensions greater than 150 mmHg
–Impairment of macrophage function
–Hypoventilation in COLD and resultant ventricular dysrhythmias secondary to rapid arterial carbon dioxide tension reduction (CO_2 narcosis)

CONTRAINDICATIONS

–Concurrent use of oxygen therapy while smoking
–Prolonged oxygen therapy greater than 50%
–Administration greater than 2½ atmospheres
–Greater than 150 mmHg arterial oxygen tension in premature infants

SPECIAL PRECAUTIONS

–COLD/COPD
–Infants

OTHER SPECIAL INFORMATION

–Cessation of grand mal seizures secondary to oxygen administration at greater than 2½ atmospheres occurs with resumption of normal air breathing.
–Humidification should accompany all forms of oxygen therapy.
–Optimal dose of oxygen concentration should be determined by the minimal amount required to reverse potentially lethal hypoxemia without producing dangerous side effects.
–Arterial blood gas samples should be taken before initiation of therapy and periodically during therapy to enable maintenance of lowest effective oxygen.
–Post No Smoking signs on patient's door and above the bed when oxygen is in use.
–Therapeutic oxygen administration is titrated to PO_2 of 60–80 mmHg. In chronic obstructive pulmonary disease, it is titrated to PO_2 of 55–60 mmHg.
–Monitor continuously patient's response to oxygen therapy including respiratory rate, depth, pattern; pulse rate, blood pressure; skin temperature and color, level of consciousness; presence of tremor.
–Ventricular dysrhythmias may indicate hypoxemia.
–With severe hypotension/cardiovascular collapse, tissue hypoxemia may be present despite adequate PO_2 levels.
–Changes in oxygen therapy are generally followed by arterial blood gas samples within 30 min to 2 hr, depending on patient's clinical response.

ANTIDOTE

SEVERE REACTIONS

–D/C drug immediately and initiate appropriate treatment for symptoms.

OTHER REACTIONS

–Notify physician of any side effects and initiate appropriate actions.

OXYTOCIN Pitocin, Syntocinon, Uteracon

CLASS

–Hormone (oxytoxic)

USES

–Initiate or improve uterine contraction during third-stage labor and overcome uterine inertia
–Induce labor in case of maternal diabetes, preeclampsia, eclampsia, erythroblastosis fetalis
–Management of inevitable, incomplete, or missed abortion
–Control of postpartum hemorrhage and promotion of postpartum uterine involution

ACTION

–Acts directly on myofibrils to produce phasic contractions associated with normal delivery and on mammary glands to stimulate lactation

USUAL DOSAGE/ROUTE

ADULT

INDUCTION OF LABOR

–IV infusion: 1 ml ampule (10 U) per liter in D_5W or NS (0.01 milliunit/ml) at 1–2 milliunits/min and may gradually increase in increments not greater than 1 milliunit/min titrated to normal contraction pattern and fetal response to a maximum of 20 milliunits/min

POSTPARTUM HEMORRHAGE

–IV infusion: 10 U in 1 liter D_5W or NS at rates adjusted to control uterine atony (approx. 10–20 milliunits/min)

–IM: 3–10 U (0.3–1.0 ml) after placental delivery

PROMOTION OF MILK LETDOWN

–Intranasal: 1 spray or 1–3 drops in 1 or both nostrils 2–3 min before breastfeeding or pumping

PEDIATRIC

–Not for use in children

ADVERSE/SIDE EFFECTS

RAPID FETAL

–Bradycardia
–Extrasystole
–Hypoxia
–Neonatal jaundice
–Intracranial hemorrhage
–Trauma secondary to rapid movement through pelvis
–Death

RAPID MOTHER

–Hypersensitivity (uterine hypertonicity, spasm, tetanic contraction, uterine rupture, anaphylaxis)
–N & V
–Postpartum hemorrhage
–Hypotension
–Extrasystoles and other dysrhythmias
–Decreased uterine blood flow
–Fatal afibrinogenemia
–Severe water intoxication leading to convulsions, coma, and death
–Cyanosis
–Anxiety
–Dyspnea

GRADUAL

–Hyponatremia
–Hypochloremia
–Thrombocytopenia
–Edema

CONTRAINDICATIONS

- –Hypersensitivity
- –Significant cephalopelvic disproportion
- –Unfavorable fetal position or presentation
- –Obstetrical emergencies where benefit/risk ratio favors surgical intervention
- –Fetal distress where delivery is not imminent
- –Prolonged use in uterine inertia or severe toxemia
- –Hypertonic uterine patterns
- –Cord prolapse
- –Placenta previa
- –Prematurity
- –History of sepsis
- –History of traumatic delivery
- –Primipara over age 35
- –Condition predisposing to thromboplastin or amniotic fluid embolism (dead fetus, abruptio placentas)
- –Previous cervical surgery or cesarean section
- –Concurrent use with CYCLOPROPANE anesthesia or vasoconstrictors

SPECIAL PRECAUTIONS

- –First and second stages of labor

OTHER SPECIAL INFORMATION

- –Never administer simultaneously by more than one route.
- –Monitor fluid intake closely, secondary to antidiuretic effects of OXYTOCIN.
- –Maternal death has occurred when used during first and second stages of labor.
- –Rotate bottle gently when diluting for IV administration to assure equal distribution in solution.
- –Document baseline data (VS, I&O, weight, fetal heart tone and rate, strength, duration, and frequency of contraction).
- –Patient should be continuously observed by qualified personnel, and a physician should be immediately available to handle complications.
- –Monitor maternal and fetal vital signs and contractions every 15 min.

–Onset of action = 1 min following IV administration, duration shorter than 1 min; onset of IM injection = 3–7 min, duration = 30–60 min.
–This drug can precipitate hypertensive crisis.
–Discontinue immediately for prolonged contractions (occurring at less than 2-min intervals) and turn patient on side.

ANTIDOTE

SEVERE REACTIONS

–D/C drug immediately and initiate appropriate treatment for symptoms.
–Treat overdose with MAGNESIUM SULFATE (10 ml of 20% solution).
–Implement ALS protocols for life-threatening dysrhythmias.

OTHER REACTIONS

–Notify physician of any side effects and initiate appropriate actions.

PANCURONIUM BROMIDE Pavulon

CLASS
–Neuromuscular blocking agent (nondepolarizing)

USES
–Facilitation of endotracheal intubation
–Skeletal muscle relaxation during mechanical ventilation, surgery, or general anesthesia

ACTION
–Prevents neuromuscular transmission by blocking the effect of acetylcholine at the myoneural junction, providing skeletal muscle paralysis
–Has no analgesic or aniolytic effects

USUAL DOSAGE/ROUTE

ADULT
–IV: 0.04–0.1 mg/kg, then 0.01 mg/kg every ½–1 hr to maintain paralysis or 0.015 mg/kg to allow mechanical ventilation

PEDIATRIC
–More than 10 yr: IV: 0.04–0.1 mg/kg, then 1/5 initial dose every ½–1 hr

ADVERSE/SIDE EFFECTS

RAPID
–Mild tachycardia
–Apnea
–Wheezing
–Burning sensation along vein
–Allergic reactions
–Bronchospasm
–Ventricular extra systoles

GRADUAL
–Weakness from prolonged skeletal muscle relaxation
–Excessive salivation in children

–Excessive sweating in children
–Rashes
–Pruritis
–Prolonged apnea

CONTRAINDICATIONS
–Hypersensitivity to bromide ion

SPECIAL PRECAUTIONS
–Pregnant or lactating patients
–Pulmonary disease
–Renal disease
–Liver impairment
–Elderly or debilitated patients
–Electrolyte disturbances
–Dehydration
–Patients receiving cardiac glycosides
–Extreme caution with myasthenia gravis or myasthenic syndromes
–Children less than 2 yr

OTHER SPECIAL INFORMATION
–Onset is 30–40 seconds after IV administration, peaks in 3–5 min.
–This drug rapidly distributes into extracellular fluid.
–This drug is excreted mostly unchanged by the kidneys.
–Store in refrigerator. Do not store in plastic containers or syringes.
–Frequently (every 2 hr) instill artificial tears and cover eyes to prevent drying of cornea.
–Monitor heart rate, ECG, and blood pressure periodically throughout drug therapy; may cause a slight increase in heart rate and blood pressure.

ANTIDOTE

SEVERE REACTIONS
–D/C drug immediately and initiate appropriate treatment for symptoms.
–Treat overdose with EDROPHONIUM or NEOSTIGMINE and

ATROPINE SULFATE. Patient may require mechanical ventilation.

OTHER REACTIONS

–Notify physician of any side effects and initiate appropriate actions.
–Monitor vital signs frequently until patient is fully recovered.

PENICILLIN G BENZATHINE Bicillin, Bicillin L-A, Megacillin, Permapen, and others

CLASS

–Broad-spectrum antibiotic (anti-infective)

USES

–Mild-to-moderate infections of the upper respiratory tract due to susceptible streptococci
–Venereal infections
–Prophylaxis for rheumatic fever and/or chorea
–Follow-up therapy for rheumatic heart disease or acute glomerulonephritis
–Otitis media
–Skin and soft tissue infections
–Pneumococcal pneumonia

ACTION

–Binds to bacterial cell wall resulting in cell death

USUAL DOSAGE/ROUTE

ADULT

–PO: 400,000–600,000 units every 4–6 hr
–IM: 1.2–2.4 million units single dose

PEDIATRIC

–PO (more than 12 yr): 400,000–600,000 units every 6–12 hr
–PO (less than 12 yr): 25,000–90,000 units/kg/day in 3–6 divided doses

–IM (less than 27 kg): 900,000 units, single dose
–IM (more than 27 kg): 300,000–600,000 units, single dose or 50,000 units/kg

ADVERSE/SIDE EFFECTS

RAPID
–NVD
–Convulsions
–Allergic reaction

GRADUAL
–Bone marrow depression
–Granulocytopenia
–Vaginitis
–Moniliasis
–Coma
–Rashes

CONTRAINDICATIONS
–Hypersensitivity to PENICILLINS or BENZATHINES
–Neonates

SPECIAL PRECAUTIONS
–Patients with significant allergies and/or asthma
–Should be used in pregnancy only if clearly needed
–Use cautiously in renal insufficiency
–Lactation
–Allergy to CEPHALOSPORINS

OTHER SPECIAL INFORMATION
–Administer to patient with an empty stomach for best absorption.
–Administer deep IM into large muscle mass.
–This drug is variably absorbed from the GI tract.
–This drug is minimally metabolized by the liver, excreted mainly unchanged by the kidneys.
–Do not inject IM dose into or near an artery or nerve.

ANTIDOTE

SEVERE REACTIONS

–D/C drug immediately and initiate appropriate treatment for symptoms.
–Treat anaphylaxis with EPINEPHRINE HCL, AMINOPHYLLINE, OXYGEN, IV corticosteroids, and other ALS procedures as indicated.

OTHER REACTIONS

–Notify physician of any side effects and initiate appropriate actions.

PENICILLIN G POTASSIUM, PENICILLIN G SODIUM Acrocillin, Burcillin-G, Deltapen, Megacillin, Pentids, Pfizerpen, Pfizerpen-G, and others

CLASS

–Broad-spectrum antibiotic (anti-infective)

USES

–Treatment of a wide variety of gram-positive and gram-negative infections including: pneumococcal pneumonia, streptococcal pharyngitis, syphilis, gonorrhea, Lyme disease, otitis media, and gingivitis
–Prophylaxis of bacterial endocarditis
–Treatment of enterococcal infections (requires the addition of an aminoglycoside)
–Prevention of rheumatic fever/chorea
–Skin and skin structure infections (staphylococcal strains)

ACTION

–Interferes with cell wall replication of susceptible organisms, causing it to become unstable and resulting in the bursting of the cell wall from the osmotic pressure changes

USUAL DOSAGE/ROUTE

ADULT (streptococcal/pneumococcal, mild-to-moderately severe)

- –PO: 200,000–500,000 U every 6–12 hr × 10 days or until afebrile × 2 days
- –IM, IV: 1,000,000–5,000,000 U every 6–8 hr

PEDIATRIC (less than 12 yr)

- –PO: 25,000–90,000 U/kg/day in 3–6 divided doses
- –IM, IV: 6,250–25,000 U/kg every 6–8 hr

NEONATES

- –IM, IV: 30,000 U/kg every 12 hr up to 1,000,000 U/day for major infections

ADVERSE/SIDE EFFECTS

RAPID

- –NVD
- –Epigastric distress
- –Phlebitis at IV site
- –Pain at IM site
- –Lethargy
- –Hallucinations
- –Coma
- –Convulsions

GRADUAL

- –Rashes
- –Hemolytic anemia
- –Bone marrow depression
- –Granulocytopenia
- –Glomerulonephritis
- –Vaginitis
- –Moniliasis
- –Black hairy tongue
- –Depression

CONTRAINDICATIONS

- –Hypersensitivity to any PENICILLIN
- –Cross-sensitivity with CEPHALOSPORINS may exist

SPECIAL PRECAUTIONS
–Pregnant or lactating patients
–Individuals with history of significant allergies and/or asthma
–Severe renal insufficiency (dosage reduction recommended)

OTHER SPECIAL INFORMATION
–This drug is best taken on an empty stomach.
–Acidic fruit juices or other acidic beverages should be avoided within one hour of administration because they interfere with absorption.
–Store in a dry, tight container.
This drug is minimally metabolized by the liver, excreted mainly unchanged by the kidneys.
–Hyperkalemia may develop following large doses of this drug.

ANTIDOTE
SEVERE REACTIONS
–D/C drug immediately and initiate appropriate treatment for symptoms.
–Treat anaphylaxis by maintaining airway, administer EPINEPHRINE, AMINOPHYLLINE.
–Administer O_2, IV corticosteroids.
OTHER REACTIONS
–Notify physician of any side effects and initiate appropriate actions.

PENTAZOCINE HCL (tablet), PENTAZOCINE LACTATE (injection) Talwin

CLASS
–Narcotic analgesic

USES
–Relief of moderate-to-severe pain associated with surgical procedures, medical disorders, and during labor

ACTION

–Binds to the opiate receptor in the CNS to alter the perception of and response to pain; analgesic effect is ⅓ to ¼ that of MORPHINE

USUAL DOSAGE/ROUTE

ADULT

–PO: 50–100 mg every 3–4 hr, not to exceed 600 mg/day
–SC, IM: 30–60 mg every 3–4 hr, not to exeed 360 mg/day
–IV: 30 mg every 3–4 hr as needed, not to exceed 360 mg/day

PEDIATRIC

–Not recommended for use in children under age 12

ADVERSE/SIDE EFFECTS

RAPID

–Vertigo
–N & V
–Tachycardia
–Sweating
–Drowsiness
–Sedation
–Headache
–Euphoria
–Rash

GRADUAL

–Urinary retention
–Formation of sterile abscesses
–Anorexia
–Constipation
–Cramps

CONTRAINDICATIONS

–Hypersensitivity
–Addiction to narcotics

SPECIAL PRECAUTIONS

–Pregnant or lactating patients
–Renal disease

–Liver disease
–Respiratory depression
–Increased intracranial pressure
–Addictive personality
–Severe heart disease
–Children less than 18 years

OTHER SPECIAL INFORMATION

–Do not mix in syringe with soluble BARBITURATES because a precipitate will form.
–Administer IV drug slowly over at least 1 min and diluted with 1 ml of sterile water for each 5 mg.
–Avoid concurrent use of alcohol and other CNS depressants.

ANTIDOTE

SEVERE REACTIONS

–D/C drug immediately and initiate appropriate treatment for symptoms.
–Reverse respiratory depression with NALOXONE 0.2–0.8 mg IV, OXYGEN, IV fluids.
–Treat hypotension with vasopressors such as DOPAMINE or METARAMINOL.

OTHER REACTIONS

–Notify physician of any side effects and initiate appropriate actions.

PHENOBARBITAL, PHENOBARBITAL SODIUM Barbita, Eskatab, Floramine, Luminol, Orpine, Solubarb, Solfoton, Stental

CLASS

–Anticonvulsant (barbiturate), sedative, hyponotic (barbiturate)

USES

- –Anticonvulsant in tonic–clonic (grand mal), partial, and febrile seizures in children
- –Sedative/hypnotic and in other situations in which sedation may be required
- –Chronic cholestasis
- –Hyperbilirubinemia
- –Insomnia

ACTION

- –Produces all levels of CNS depression
- –Depresses the sensory cortex, decreases motor activity, alters cerebellar function, and raises the seizure threshold at the cerebral cortex
- –Capable of inducing (speeding up) enzymes in the liver that metabolize drugs, bilirubin, and other compounds

USUAL DOSAGE/ROUTE

ADULT (sedation)

–PO, IM: 30–120 mg/day in 2–3 divided doses

ADULT (anticonvulsant)

–PO: 100–300 mg/day, single dose or 2–3 divided doses

–IV: 200–600 mg (total of 600 mg/24-hr period)

ADULT (status epilepticus)

–IV: 10–20 mg/kg, administered by IV infusion, should run no faster than 50 mg/min

ADULT (hypnotic)

–PO: 100–320 mg at bedtime

–SC, IM, IV: 100–325 mg at bedtime

PEDIATRIC (sedation)

–PO: 2–6 mg/kg/day in 3 divided doses

PEDIATRIC (anticonvulsant)

–PO: 3–5 mg/kg/day, single dose or divided dose

–IV: 100–400 mg

PEDIATRIC (status epilepticus)

–IV: 5–20 mg/kg, should begin with 5–10 mg/kg, may repeat every 10–15 min, up to 20 mg/kg, run no faster than 50 mg/min

PEDIATRIC (hypnotic)
–SC, IM, IV: 3–5 mg/kg at bedtime

ADVERSE/SIDE EFFECTS

RAPID
–Rash
–Headache
–Flushing
–Vertigo
–Drowsiness
–Respiratory depression
–Laryngospasm (IV only)
–Hypotension (IV only)
–N & V
–Stimulation
–Coma

GRADUAL
–Neuralgia
–Hangover
–Stevens–Johnson syndrome

CONTRAINDICATIONS
–Hypersensitivity to barbiturates
–Marked impairment of liver function
–Respiratory disease in which dyspnea or obstruction is evident
–Nephritis
–Hyperthyroidism
–Diabetes mellitus
–Pregnancy
–Lactation
–Uncontrolled severe pain

SPECIAL PRECAUTIONS
–Patients who may be suicidal or who may have been addicted to drugs previously
–Elderly patients (dosage reduction recommended)
–Anemia

OTHER SPECIAL INFORMATION

–This drug is metabolized by the liver, excreted by kidneys.
–Monitor respiratory status, pulse, and blood pressure frequently during IV administration.
–Serum PHENOBARBITAL levels should be routinely monitored when used as an anticonvulsant. Therapeutic levels are 10–40 mcg/ml.
–Advise patient to take medication exactly as prescribed.
–Advise patients not to discontinue medication without consulting physician. Abrupt withdrawal may precipitate seizures or status epilepticus.
–Chronic use may lead to dependence.
–Use with MAO inhibitors may prolong the effects of barbiturates.

ANTIDOTE

SEVERE REACTIONS

–D/C drug immediately and initiate appropriate treatment for symptoms.
–Treat overdose with IV CALCIUM GLUCONATE.

OTHER REACTIONS

–Notify physician of any side effects and initiate appropriate actions.

PHENTOLAMINE MESYLATE Regitine, Rogitine

CLASS

–Alpha-adrenergic blocking agent (antihypertensive)

USES

–Hypertension associated with pheochromocytoma or adrenergic excess, such as administration of PHENYLEPHRINE HCL or CLONODINE withdrawal
–Control of blood pressure during surgical removal of pheochromocytoma

–Treatment or prevention of dermal necrosis following extravasation or NOREPINEPHRINE, PHENYCEPHRINE, or DOPAMINE
–Indicated for the diagnosis of pheomocytoma by the Regitine blocking test

ACTION

–Produces an alpha-adrenergic block of relatively short duration that dilates peripheral blood vessels, lowers peripheral resistance, resulting in lowered blood pressure

USUAL DOSAGE/ROUTE

ADULT (treatment of hypertensive episode with pheochromocytoma and during surgery)
–IM, IV: 5 mg (may repeat if necessary)

ADULT (treatment/prevention of dermal necrosis)
–5–10 mg/10 ml NS injected into area of NOREPINEPHRINE/PHENYLEPHRINE/DOPAMINE extravasation within 12 hr (10 mg/1000 ml NOREPINEPHRINE solution is preventive dose)

ADULT (pheochromocytoma)
–IM, IV: 5 mg (may be given IM, but IV is preferred)

PEDIATRIC (hypertensive episode with pheochromocytoma and during surgery)
–IV, IM: 1 mg or 0.1 mg/kg or 3 mg/M^2 given 1–2 hr preop, may be repeated if necessary

PEDIATRIC (pheochromocytoma)
–IV: 1 mg or 3 mg/M^2 or 0.1 mg/kg
–IM: 3 mg

ADVERSE/SIDE EFFECTS

RAPID
–Dry mouth
–NVD
–Abdominal pain
–Hypotension
–Tachycardia
–Angina

–Dysrhythmias
–Dizziness
–MI

GRADUAL
–Weakness
–Nasal congestion

CONTRAINDICATIONS
–Hypersensitivity
–Coronary and cerebral arteriosclerosis
–Renal impairment
–MI
–Angina

SPECIAL PRECAUTIONS
–Pregnant or lactating patients
–Peptic ulcer disease
–Ederly patients (more susceptible to hypotensive effects; dosage reduction recommended)

OTHER SPECIAL INFORMATION
–Monitor blood pressure, pulse, and ECG every 2 min until stable during IV administration.
–Patient should remain supine throughout parenteral administration.
–This drug is metabolized in liver, excreted in urine.
–Do not mix in the syringe with any other drug except LEVARTERENOL.

ANTIDOTE

SEVERE REACTIONS
–D/C drug immediately and initiate appropriate treatment for symptoms.
–Treat overdose with vasopressor such as NOREPINEPHRINE.

OTHER REACTIONS
–Notify physician of any side effects and initiate appropriate actions.

PHENYLEPHRINE HCL Neo-Synephrine

CLASS
–Adrenergic (nasal decongestant), vasopressor

USES
–Hypotension
–Paroxysmal supraventricular tachycardia
–Shock
–Topically for symptomatic relief of rhinitis of common cold, allergic rhinitis, and sinusitis; mydriation during ophthalmoscopic examination or surgery to temporarily relieve eye irritation

ACTION
–Strong alpha-adrenergic cardiac stimulator producing elevation in systolic and diastolic pressures by constriction of arterioles leading to reflex decrease in heart rate
–Vasoconstriction and short mydriasis produced by topical eye application; intraocular pressure reduced by increased outflow and decreased rate of aqueous humor secretion
–Nasal decongestant action, produced by vasoconstriction of arterioles

USUAL DOSAGE/ROUTE

ADULT
–SC, IM: 1–10 mg (initial dose not to exceed 5 mg) and may repeat every 10–15 min if needed
–IV: 0.1–0.6 mg (initial dose not to exceed 0.5 mg) and may repeat every 10–15 min if needed
–IV infusion: 10 mg/500 ml D_5W given at 100–180 gtts/min, then 40–60 gtts/min titrated to BP
–Ophthalmic: 0.5% jelly
–Nasal: 0.25–1.0% in each nostril every 3–4 hr

PEDIATRIC (under 6 yr)
–SC, IM: 0.1 mg/kg
–Ophthalmic: 0.5% jelly

PEDIATRIC (over 6 yr)
–Nasal: 0.25% in each nostril every 3–4 hr

PEDIATRIC (infants)
–Nasal: 0.125–0.2% in each nostril every 2–4 hr

ADVERSE/SIDE EFFECTS

RAPID (SYSTEMIC USE)
–Tachycardia
–Palpitations
–Extrasystole
–Hypertension
–Dizziness
–Light-headedness
–Weakness
–Fullness in head
–Trembling
–Tingling of extremities
–Sweating
–Pallor
–N & V
–Cardiac dysrhythmias

NASAL USE
–Burning
–Stinging
–Drying
–Sneezing

OPHTHALMIC USE
–Transient stinging
–Conjunctival allergy
–Headache
–Blurred vision

GRADUAL
–Sleeplessness
–Tissue necrosis
–Gangrene
–Rebound congestion (nasal)

CONTRAINDICATIONS
–Hypersensitivity to this or other adrenergic drugs
–Hypertension
–Severe coronary artery disease
–Ventricular fibrillation
–Narrow-angle glaucoma
–Pheochromocytoma
–Concurrent use of tricyclic antidepressants, MAO inhibitors, and OXYTOXIC drugs
–Bradycardia
–Cerebral arteriosclerosis
–Hyperthyroidism
–HALOTHANE anesthesia
–Respiratory obstruction, asthma particularly

SPECIAL PRECAUTIONS
–Pregnant or lactating patients
–Embolism
–Peripheral vascular disease
–Diabetes mellitus

OTHER SPECIAL INFORMATION
–Continued, frequent use of higher concentrations of topical decongestants will produce rebound congestion.
–Use topical decongestants sparingly and only at recommended dosages, particularly in children and the elderly.
–Continuous IV infusion rate is prescribed by the physician (usually initial rate of 100–180 drops/min for shock, decreasing to 40–60 drops/min as blood pressure stabilizes).
–Clear nasal passages before nasal administration.

ANTIDOTE

SEVERE REACTIONS
–D/C drug immediately and initiate appropriate treatment for symptoms.
–Treat hypertension with antihypertensive such as PHENTOLAMINE.
–Treat topical mydriatic reaction with LEVODOPA.
–Treat overdose with NOREPINEPHRINE.

OTHER REACTIONS

–Notify physician of any side effects and initiate appropriate actions.

PHENYTOIN SODIUM Dilantin, Diphen, Diphenylan, Diphenylhydantoin, DPH

CLASS

–Anticonvulsant, antidysrhythmic

USES

–Grand mal and psychomotor seizures
–Nonepileptic seizures associated with Reye's syndrome or after head trauma
–Trigeminal neuralgia
–Bell's palsy
–Ventricular dysrhythmias unresponsive to LIDOCAINE or PROCAINAMIDE
–Supraventricular and ventricular dysrhythmias induced by cardiac glycosides

ACTION

–Decreases excitability of myocardial cells
–Exerts a selective action on the cerebral cortex of the brain, raising its threshold to stimuli

USUAL DOSAGE/ROUTE

ADULT (anticonvulsant)

–PO: Loading dose 900 mg–1.5 gm divided 3 times/day (maintenance dose 300 mg daily)
–IV: Loading dose 900 mg–1.5 gm at 50 mg/min

ADULT (antidysrhythmic)

–PO: Loading dose 1 gm divided over 24 hr, followed by 500 mg daily for 2 days, then maintenance dose 300 mg daily

–IV: 250 mg over 5 min until dysrhythmias subside or until 1 gm has been given

PEDIATRIC (anticonvulsant)

–PO: Loading dose 15 mg/kg divided every 8–12 hr, then 5–7 mg/kg every 12 hr

–IV: Loading dose 15 mg/kg at 50 mg/min

PEDIATRIC (antidysrhythmic)

–PO: Loading dose 15 mg/kg divided 3 times/day, maintenance dose of 3–8 mg/kg divided 2 times/day, not to exceed 300 mg

–IV: 3–8 mg/kg given over several minutes

ADVERSE/SIDE EFFECTS

RAPID

–Hypotension
–N & V
–Skin rash
–Exfoliative dermatitis
–Stevens–Johnson syndrome
–Toxic epidermal necrolysis

GRADUAL

–Ataxia
–Slurred speech
–Confusion
–Nystagmus
–Mental dullness
–Blood dyscrasias
–Diplopia
–Aplastic anemia
–Agranulocytosis
–Hepatic damage
–Gum hyperplasia (with chronic ingestion)

CONTRAINDICATIONS

–Hypersensitivity
–Psychiatric disease
–Bradycardia (sinoatrial and atrioventricular)
–Heart block
–Pregnancy

SPECIAL PRECAUTIONS
–Liver disease
–Renal disease

OTHER SPECIAL INFORMATION
–With IV administration, give slowly IV push not exceeding 50 mg/min.
–Flush IV tubing with NS before and after IV administration, will precipitate with D_5W.
–Use only clear solution for IV administration.
–Therapeutic serum level is 10–20 mcg/ml.
–Use of alcohol may diminish drug's action.
–Give PO doses with food to decrease GI side effects.
–Monitor EKG if giving drug for dysrhythmias.
–Numerous drug interactions, see AHFS 28:12.

ANTIDOTE
SEVERE REACTIONS
–D/C drug immediately and initiate appropriate treatment for symptoms.
OTHER REACTIONS
–Notify physician of any side effects and initiate appropriate actions.

PHYTONADIONE (Vitamin K_1) Aqua Mephyton, Konakion, Mephyton

CLASS
–Vitamin K_1 (fat-soluble vitamin)

USES
–Antidote for WARFARIN SODIUM
–Hypoprothrombinemia
–Prevention of hypoprothrombinemia caused by oral anticoagulants
–Vitamin K malabsorption syndromes

–Prophylaxis of hypoprothrombinemia of the newborn
–Certain forms of liver disease
–Ulcerative colitis
–Obstructive jaundice

ACTION
–Is essential to the synthesis of prothrombin by the liver and adequate blood clotting (factors II, VII, IX, X)

USUAL DOSAGE/ROUTE

ADULT
–PO, IM, SC: 2.5–10 mg repeated in 12–48 hr with continued high prothrombin time up to 25 mg

PEDIATRIC
–IM, SC (more than 1 yr): 5–10 mg single dose
–IM; SC (less than 1 yr): 1–2 mg single dose

ADVERSE/SIDE EFFECTS

RAPID
–Pain, edema at injection site
–Flushing sensation
–Tachycardia
–Weak pulse
–Brief hypotension
–Profuse sweating
–Unusual taste
–Dyspnea

GRADUAL
–Dizziness
–Gastric upset
–Hemolytic anemia

CONTRAINDICATIONS
–Hypersensitivity to drug
–Hepatic disease

SPECIAL PRECAUTIONS
–Pregnancy
–Impaired liver function

OTHER SPECIAL INFORMATION

–Vitamin K_1 is extremely light sensitive.
–IM, SC onset = 1–2 hr; peak = 3–6 hr; duration = 12–14 hr.
–IV use should be limited due to high incidence of anaphylaxis and death.
–Frequent determinations of prothrombin time for decrease back to normal are essential.
–In treatment of oral anticoagulant-induced prothrombin deficiency, lowest possible dose should be used so that refractoriness to further anticoagulant therapy is minimized.
–Administration of whole blood or plasma may also be required in severe bleeding because of the delayed onset on this drug.
–Teach patient to include foods containing vitamin K_1 in his/her diet during therapy, including beef liver, spinach, tomatoes, coffee, asparagus, broccoli, cabbage, lettuce, greens, dairy products, and not to alter diet drastically while on this drug.

ANTIDOTE

SEVERE REACTIONS

–D/C drug immediately and initiate appropriate treatment for symptoms.

OTHER REACTIONS

–Notify physician of any side effects and initiate appropriate actions.

PINDOLOL Visken

CLASS

–Beta-adrenergic blocker (antihypertensive, peripheral vasodilator)

USES

–Moderate-to-severe hypertension not responsive to other therapy

–May be used topically to treat alopecia

ACTION

–Blocks stimulation of beta-1 (myocardial), and beta-2 (pulmonary) receptor sites to lower heart rate and blood pressure

USUAL DOSAGE/ROUTE

ADULT

–PO: 5–10 mg 2 times a day, increasing by 10 mg/day every 3–4 weeks to a max of 60 mg/day

PEDIATRIC

–Safe use in children not established

ADVERSE/SIDE EFFECTS

RAPID

–NVD
–Rash
–Bronchospasm
–Dyspnea

GRADUAL

–Hypotension
–Bradycardia
–Insomnia
–Visual changes/double vision
–Dizziness
–Anxiety
–Fatigue
–Edema
–Chest pain
–Claudication
–AV block
–Ischemic colitis
–Abdominal pain
–Alopecia

–Fever
–Agranulocytosis
–Thrombocytopenia
–Impotence
–Joint pain
–Muscle pain

CONTRAINDICATIONS
–Hypersensitivity
–Cardiogenic shock
–2nd- or 3rd-degree heart block
–Bradycardia
–Bronchiospastic disease
–CHF/PE
–Hypotension
–COPD
–Asthma

SPECIAL PRECAUTIONS
–Pregnant or lactating patients
–Diabetes mellitus (masks hypoglycemia)
–Renal disease (requires reduced dosage)
–Thyroid disease
–Major surgery
–CAD
–Children

OTHER SPECIAL INFORMATION
–The antihypertensive effect usually occurs in approximately 7 days and may last up to 2 weeks.
–Assess vital signs prior to therapy and periodically during therapy for decreases.
–Perform daily weights to assess for fluid retention.
–Do not discontinue abruptly.
–This drug may lower blood glucose levels and mask signs of hypoglycemia in diabetic patients.

ANTIDOTE

SEVERE REACTIONS

–D/C drug immediately and initiate appropriate treatment for symptoms.

–Treat bradycardia with IV ATROPINE SULFATE.

–Treat hypotension with an IV vasopressor such as DOPAMINE or METARAMINOL.

–Treat bronchospasm with IV THEOPHYLLINE.

–Treat dysrhythmias with an IV cardiac glycoside such as DIGOXIN.

OTHER REACTIONS

–Notify physician of any side effects and initiate appropriate actions.

PLASMA PROTEIN FRACTION Plasmanate, Plasma-Plex, Plasmatein, Protenate

CLASS

–Plasma volume expander (blood derivative)

USES

–Maintain cardiac output in circulatory volume deficiencies such as hypovolemic shock, hemorrhage, burns, hypoproteinemia

ACTION

–Provides colloidal oncotic pressure similar to human plasma, causing the shift of water from extravascular tissues into the intravascular space and expanding blood volume

USUAL DOSAGE/ROUTE

ADULT

–*Hypovolemic shock:* IV infusion: 250–500 ml (12.5–25 gms protein), not to exceed 10 ml/min

–*Hypoproteinemia:* IV infusion: 1000–1500 ml (50–75 gms protein), not to exceed 8 ml/min

PEDIATRIC
–IV infusion: 22–33 ml/kg at 5–10 ml/min

ADVERSE/SIDE EFFECTS

RAPID
–N & V
–Rash
–Urticaria
–Flushing
–Dyspnea
–Irregular pulse

GRADUAL
–Increased salivation
–Fever and chills
–Headache
–Paresthesias
–Cyanosis in pulmonary overload
–Pulmonary edema
–Fluid overload
–Hypotension
–Back pain

CONTRAINDICATIONS

–Hypersensitivity to albumin
–Severe anemia
–CHF
–Increased intravascular volume
–Cardiopulmonary bypass procedures

SPECIAL PRECAUTIONS

–Severe liver disease
–Severe renal disease
–Dehydration
–Decreased cardiac reserve
–Pregnant patients

OTHER SPECIAL INFORMATION

–Too rapid infusion may cause blood pressure changes, either hypotension or hypertension.

–Large doses should be avoided to prevent anemia.
–This drug is incompatible with any solution containing alcohol or with NOREPINEPHRINE.
–May administer this drug undiluted, or may dilute with NS or D_5W.

ANTIDOTE

SEVERE REACTIONS

–D/C drug immediately and initiate appropriate treatment for symptoms.

OTHER REACTIONS

–Notify physician of any side effects and initiate appropriate actions.
–If reaction occurs, use a new lot if therapy reinstated.

POTASSIUM ACETATE, POTASSIUM BICARBONATE, POTASSIUM CHLORIDE, POTASSIUM GLUCONATE, POTASSIUM PHOSPHATE K-Ciel, K-Lor, Klotrix, K-Lyte, Micro-K, Slow-K, and others

CLASS

–Potassium supplement (electrolyte)

USES

–Prevention and treatment of potassium deficiency that may occur with severe vomiting, diarrhea, diabetic ketoacidosis, intestinal drainage or malabsorption, prolonged diuresis, metabolic alkalosis
–Treatment of cardiac dysrhythmias particularly associated with use of digitalis glycosides
–Treatment of Ménière's disease

ACTION

–The principal cation necessary for maintenance of intracellular tonicity, transmission of nerve impulses, contraction of cardiac, skeletal, and smooth muscles, and maintenance of normal renal function

USUAL DOSAGE/ROUTE

ADULT

–*Prevention:* PO: 20–50 meq/day in 3–4 divided doses;
–*Treatment of depletion:* PO: 40–100 mEq/day in 3–4 divided doses
–IV: Not to exceed 20 mEq/hr up to 150 mEq/day (concentration = 40 mEq/liter)

PEDIATRIC

–PO, IV: 2–3 mEq/kg/day or 40 mEq/M^2/day in 3–4 divided doses

ADVERSE/SIDE EFFECTS

RAPID

–Dysrhythmias
–EKG changes
–NVD
–Abdominal pain
–Bleeding at injection site

GRADUAL

–Hyperkalemia (mental confusion, listlessness, muscle weakness, paresthesia of extremities, respiratory distress, hypotension, cardiac dysrhythmias, heart block, cardiac arrest, altered sensitivity to digitalis glycoside)

CONTRAINDICATIONS

–Hypersensitivity
–Hyperkalemia
–Severe renal insufficiency with oliguria, anuria, azotemia
–Severe tissue trauma
–Severe hemolytic reaction
–Untreated Addison's disease
–Heat cramps
–Concurrent administration of aldosterone antagonists or TRIAMTERENE
–Digitalis intoxication in presence of conduction disturbances

SPECIAL PRECAUTIONS
–ASPIRIN allergy
–Cardiac disease
–Renal impairment
–Diabetes mellitus (liquids contain sugar)
–GI hypomotility
–Dysphagia

OTHER SPECIAL INFORMATION
–For critical IV infusion, a saline solution may be used unless contraindicated because dextrose fluids may decrease serum K^+ levels.
–Oral doses should be diluted per package instructions in water or citrus juices, usually 4 oz/20 mEq.
–Do not administer this drug IM, SC, or IV bolus.
–Carefully monitor IV infusion to prevent fatal side effects and extravasation.
–Strictly monitor intake/output; notify physician of sudden or gradual decrease in output.
–Serial ECGs are necessary as serum potassium lows are not accurate indicators of intracellular K^+ concentrations.
–On ECG, hyperkalemia produces tall, peaked T waves.
–Hypokalemia associated with metabolic acidosis should be treated with POTASSIUM BICARBONATE, POTASSIUM CITRATE, or POTASSIUM ACETATE.
–Teach patient to add K^+ rich foods to diet after discontinuation of this drug (i.e., bananas, orange juice, avocados, whole grains, broccoli, carrots, prunes, cocoa).

ANTIDOTE

SEVERE REACTIONS
–D/C drug immediately and initiate appropriate treatment for symptoms.
–Treat acidosis with SODIUM BICARBONATE.
–Treat overdose with DEXTROSE and INSULIN to facilitate passage of the drug into the cells, and KAYEXALATE enema to remove excess K^+.

OTHER REACTIONS
–Notify physician of any side effects and initiate appropriate actions.

–Treat EKG effects with CARDIAC GLYCOSIDES or CALCIUM SALTS.

PRAZOSIN HCL Minipress

CLASS
–Antihypertensive (alpha-adrenergic blocker)

USES
–Hypertension
–CHF

ACTION
–Inhibits alpha-adrenergic receptors, causing arterial and venous dilation, reducing peripheral vascular resistance and lowering blood pressure

USUAL DOSAGE/ROUTE
ADULT
–PO: 1 mg 2–3 times/day, gradually increasing to a max of 20 mg daily (maintenance is 6–15 mg/day in 3 divided doses)

PEDIATRIC
–Safe use in children not established

ADVERSE/SIDE EFFECTS
RAPID
–NVD
–Rash
–Urticaria
–Dizziness
–Hypotension
–Headache
–Dry mouth
–Palpitations
–Syncope (with first dose)

–Weakness
–Light-headedness
–Unconsciousness

GRADUAL

–Drowsiness
–Fluid retention
–Depression
–Orthostatic hypotension
–Blurred vision
–Abdominal cramps
–Priapism
–Impotence

CONTRAINDICATIONS

–Hypersensitivity
–Pregnant or lactating patients

SPECIAL PRECAUTIONS

–Elderly (require reduced dosage)
–Chronic renal failure
–Liver disease
–In conjunction with other antihypertensives

OTHER SPECIAL INFORMATION

–The first dose should be given at bedtime to avoid first-dose syncope, dizziness, weakness, light-headedness, which is very common with this drug.
–Antihypertensive effect begins in approximately 2 hr, and peak = 2–4 hr (full effect may take 4–6 weeks).
–This drug potentiates the effects of other antihypertensives especially PROPRANOLOL and other beta-blockers.
–Chronic use of this drug may cause a transient fall in WBC counts, and an increase in serum BUN and uric acid levels.
–The effects of this drug are most pronounced in the diastolic blood pressure.
–Do not discontinue this drug abruptly; it may cause severe rebound hypertension.

ANTIDOTE

SEVERE REACTIONS

–D/C drug immediately and initiate appropriate treatment for symptoms.

–Treat overdose with gastric lavage or induced emesis and give activated charcoal, then treat symptomatically.

OTHER REACTIONS

–Notify physician of any side effects and initiate appropriate actions.

PREDNISONE Deltasone, Deltra, Meticorten, Panasol, Paracort, Sterapred, and others

CLASS

–Adrenocortical steroid (glucocorticoid, intermediate acting)

USES

–Replacement therapy in adrenocortical insufficiency

–Suppression of undesirable inflammatory or immune response

–In nonadrenal disease, to cause temporary remission

–In diagnostic testing, to prevent ACTH production

–Specific uses include collagen diseases, pemphigus, alopecia areata, shock not responsive to conventional therapy, ophthalmic inflammatory diseases, neoplastic disease, metastatic mammary carcinoma, allergic states, chronic ulcerative colitis, nephrotic syndrome

ACTION

–Acts at the tissue and cellular level to produce primarily glucocorticoid effects (anti-inflammatory, immunosuppressive) as well as mineralocorticoid effects (sodium retention and potassium excretion, preservation of normal water distribution, ability to excrete water load normally, and ACTH suppression)

USUAL DOSAGE/ROUTE

ADULT

–PO: 2.5–15 mg daily in 2–4 divided doses to produce desired clinical response, then decrease every 4–5 days to lowest effective dosage, usually 2.5–15 mg every day or every other day

PEDIATRIC

–PO: 0.14–2 mg/kg/day in 4 divided doses gradually decreased to 1.5 mg/kg/day after 2–3 weeks

ADVERSE/SIDE EFFECTS

RAPID

–NVD
–Convulsions
–Anaphylaxis

GRADUAL

–Fluid and electrolyte disturbance (sodium retention, calcium and potassium loss, hypokalemia alkalosis)
–Hypertension
–Thrombophlebitis
–Congestive heart failure
–Muscle weakness
–Loss of muscle mass
–Osteoporosis
–Pathologic fracture
–Septic ulcer
–Abdominal distention
–Pancreatitis
–Ulcerative esophagitis
–Impaired wound healing
–Thin fragile skin
–Hirsutism
–Acneform eruption
–Allergic dermatitis
–Urticaria
–Increased intracranial pressure with papilledema
–Vertigo
–Headache

–Syncope
–Insomnia
–Aggravation of preexisting psychiatric disorders
–Mood swings and depression
–Menstrual irregularities
–Development of cushingoid state
–Growth suppression in children
–Sterility
–Decreased glucose tolerance
–Manifestation of latent diabetes mellitus
–Subcapsular cataracts
–Glaucoma
–Increased intraocular pressure
–Exophthalmus
–Negative nitrogen balance secondary to protein catabolism
–Hyperglycemia
–Glycosuria
–Aggravation or masking of infection
–Renal calculi
–Obesity

CONTRAINDICATIONS
–Hypersensitivity
–Active or latent peptic ulcer disease
–Psychoses
–Systemic fungal infections
–Acute glomerulonephritis
–Viral skin disease
–History of or active tuberculosis
–Cushing's syndrome
–Infections uncontrolled by antibiotics
–Ocular herpes simplex
–Myasthenia gravis
–Liver disease
–Renal disease
–Cardiovascular disease
–Circulatory impairment
–Glaucoma
–Osteoporosis

–Diverticulitis
–Nonspecific ulcerative colitis

SPECIAL PRECAUTIONS

–Chronic treatment
–Pregnancy and lactation
–Children
–Depression

OTHER SPECIAL INFORMATION

–Never abruptly discontinue.
–Administer after meals and at bedtime.
–Use cautiously in children.
–Monitor weight daily; report if greater than 5 lb/week gain.
–Be alert for signs indicating potassium deficit (muscle weakness, nausea, anorexia, paresthesia, depression, postural hypotension).
–Protect from light and air in dark, tightly sealed container.
–Because of skin test suppression by PREDNISONE, testing for tuberculosis before therapy is necessary.
–Higher doses are necessary during stress.
–Continuous monitoring of blood pressure, I&O, and sleep pattern is important to recognize early complications.
–Avoid overuse of inflamed joints in which symptomatic relief is obtained with this drug.
–Abrupt withdrawal produces exacerbation of inflammatory process and adrenal insufficiency.
–Increases requirements of INSULIN and oral hypoglycemic agents in diabetes mellitus.
–Alters response to COUMADIN anticoagulants with concomitant use.
–Use cautiously with K^+-depleting diuretics.

ANTIDOTE

SEVERE REACTIONS

–D/C drug immediately and initiate appropriate treatment for symptoms.

OTHER REACTIONS

–Notify physician of any side effects and initiate appropriate actions.

PROBENECID Benemid, Benn, Benuryl, Probalan, Probenimead, Robenecid

CLASS
–Uricosuric (antigout agent; sulfonamide derivative)

USES
–Hyperuricemia in gouty arthritis
–With PENICILLINS and CEPHALOSPORINS when elevated and prolonged levels of antibiotic are indicated

ACTION
–Promotes the elimination of uric acids by the kidneys
–Renal tubular blocking agent
–Increases plasma levels of PENICILLIN and CEPHALOSPORINS by decreasing renal tubular secretion

USUAL DOSAGE/ROUTE
ADULT
–PO: 250 mg 2 times a day for 1 week, then 500 mg 2–4 times a day not to exceed 2 gms/day

PEDIATRIC (3–14 yr)
–PO: 25 mg/kg initially, then 40 mg/kg 3–4 times a day

ADVERSE/SIDE EFFECTS
RAPID
–NVD
–Hypotension
–Bradycardia
–Apnea
–Irregular respirations

GRADUAL
–Headache
–Dizziness
–Flushing
–Abdominal discomfort
–Anorexia

–Hemolytic anemia
–Dermatitis
–Fever
–Sweating
–Uric acid kidney stones (rare)
–Thirst
–Glycosuria
–Hypokalemia
–Hyperchloremia
–Hyperglycemia

CONTRAINDICATIONS
–Hypersensitivity to drug or sulfa drugs
–Blood dyscrasias
–Severe liver disease
–Uric acid kidney stones
–Severe renal disease
–Creatinine clearance less than 50 mg/min

SPECIAL PRECAUTIONS
–Pregnant or lactating patients
–Severe respiratory disease
–Cardiac edema
–Children less than 2 yr

OTHER SPECIAL INFORMATION
–Inform patient to drink increased amounts of water to maintain daily urine output of at least 2 liters.
–This drug is not useful during an acute attack of gout and may precipitate acute gouty arthritis.
–COLBENEMID is a combination tablet of 500 mg of PROBENECID and 0.5 mg of COLCHICINE (an antigout alkaloid agent).
–ASPIRIN antagonizes uricosuric activity.
–False positive glycosuria occurs when using Benedict's, Clinitest, or Feeling's solution, but not with Testape or Clinistix.

ANTIDOTE

SEVERE REACTIONS

–D/C drug immediately and initiate appropriate treatment for symptoms.

OTHER REACTIONS

–Notify physician of any side effects and initiate appropriate actions.

PROCAINAMIDE HCL Procan SR, Promaine, Pronestyl, Rhythmin, Sub-Quin

CLASS

–Antidysrhythmic

USES

–Treatment of premature ventricular contractions, ventricular tachycardia, ventricular fibrillation resistant to defibrillation, atrial fibrillation, atrial flutter, and paroxysmal atrial tachycardia

–Second-degree heart block, type I dysrhythmias

ACTION

–Depresses myocardial excitability, and delays conduction in the atrium, the bundle of His, and the ventricles (prolonged atrial refractory period much greater than ventricular)

–Anticholinergic stimulation (increased heart rate) in absence of dysrhythmias

USUAL DOSAGE/ROUTE

ADULT

–PO (Loading dose): 12 mg/kg

–PO (Maintenance dose): 6 mg/kg every 3 hr to maintain therapeutic plasma levels of 3–10 mcg/mg

–*Ventricular tachycardia:* PO: 1 gm initially followed by 50 mg/kg/day every 3 hr in equally divided doses

–*Premature ventricular contractions:* PO: 50 mg/kg/day every 3 hr in equally divided doses
–*Atrial dysrhythmias:* PO: 1.0–1.25 gm initially followed by 0.75 gm in 1 hr. If no ECG changes occur, 0.5–1.0 gm may be given every 2 hr until dysrhythmia interrupted or tolerance limit reached; maintenance is 0.5–1.0 gm every 4–6 hr
–IM: 0.5–1.0 gm every 4–8 hr
–IV bolus: 100 mg every 5 min at rate of 20 mg/min not to exceed 50 mg/min until dysrhythmia suppressed, hypotension develops, QRS complex widens by 50% of original width, or a total of 1 gm has been injected
–IV infusion: initially 500–600 mg at a constant rate over 25–30 min; maintenance: continuous infusion at 2–6 mg/min

PEDIATRIC
–PO: 50 mg/kg/24 hr (1.5 gm/M^2/24 hr) divided every 4–6 hr
–IV: 2 mg/kg/dose slowly

ADVERSE/SIDE EFFECTS

RAPID
–Hypotension
–Flushing
–Widened QRS interval
–Giddiness
–Ventricular conduction disturbances
–Muscle and joint pain
–Angioneurotic edema
–Rash
–Heart block
–Arrest

GRADUAL
–NVD
–Anorexia
–Urticaria
–Pruritus
–Systemic lupus erythematosus-like reaction
–Coombs positive hemolytic anemia
–Fever, chills

–Abdominal pain
Acute hepatomegaly
–Weakness
–Mental depression
–Psychosis with hallucinations
–Agranulocytosis

CONTRAINDICATIONS

–Hypersensitivity
–Cross-sensitivity to PROCAINE and related drugs
–Complete AV block
–Second- and third-degree AV block unless pacemaker operative
–Following electrocardioversion to sinus rhythm
–Hypotension
–Dysrhythmias secondary to digitalis toxicity or electrolyte imbalance
–MI
–Coronary occlusion

SPECIAL PRECAUTIONS

–Pregnant and lactating patients
–Children
–Renal disease
–Liver disease
–CHF
–Respiratory depression
–Myasthenia gravis

OTHER SPECIAL INFORMATION

–Do not discontinue without physician instruction.
–Monitor vital signs and ECG continuously during IV administration; serial ECG should be taken with all administration forms.
–Monitor blood count to assess for development of agranulocytosis (decreased leukocytes).
–Notify physician immediately of soreness of the mouth, throat, or gums; unexplained fever; symptoms of upper respiratory tract infection; joint pain or stiffness.
–May elevate SGOT.

–Plasma levels of 8–16 mcg/ml are potentially toxic; greater than 16 mcg/ml usually associated with toxic symptoms; monitor plasma levels frequently.
–Correction of atrial fibrillation may dislodge emboli.
–IV, IM dose peaks within 15–60 min; oral peaks 30–90 min; plasma half-life 1.5–3.0 hr.

ANTIDOTE

SEVERE REACTIONS

–D/C drug immediately and initiate appropriate treatment for symptoms.
–Treat overdose with ALS protocols as appropriate.

OTHER REACTIONS

–Notify physician of any side effects and initiate appropriate actions.

PROCAINE HCL Novocaine, Unicaine

CLASS

–Local anesthetic

USES

–Spinal anesthesia
–Epidural
–Peripheral nerve block
–Perineum
–Lower extremities

ACTION

–Stabilizes the neuronal membrane and prevents the initiation and transmission of nerve impulses

USUAL DOSAGE/ROUTE

ADULT AND PEDIATRIC (12 yr or older)

–Available in 1%, 2%, and 10% injection concentrations
–The dosage varies and depends upon the area to be an-

esthetized, the vascularity of the tissues, the number of neuronal segments to be blocked, individual tolerance, and the technique of anesthesia
–The usual rate of injection is 1 ml per 5 seconds. Full anesthesia and fixation usually occur in 5 min.

ADVERSE/SIDE EFFECTS

RAPID
–Convulsions
–Loss of consciousness
–Cardiac arrest
–Dysrhythmias
–Myocardial depression
–Tinnitus
–N & V
–Respiratory arrest
–Anaphylaxis
–Blurred vision
–Hypotension
–Pupil constriction
–Status asthmaticus

GRADUAL
–Tissue necrosis
–Cutaneous lesions
–Postspinal headache

CONTRAINDICATIONS
–Hypersensitivity
–Children less than 12 yr
–Elderly
–Severe liver disease
–Generalized septicemia

SPECIAL PRECAUTIONS
–Pregnancy
–Elderly
–Severe drug allergies

OTHER SPECIAL INFORMATION

- Assess BP, pulse, respirations during treatment.
- Monitor fetal heart tones if used during labor.
- Administer only drugs that are noncloudy and do not contain precipitates.
- Only drugs without preservatives should be used for epidural or caudal anesthesia.
- Monitor ECG for dysrhythmias during anesthesia; onset = 2–5 min; duration = 1 hr.

ANTIDOTE

SEVERE REACTIONS

- D/C drug immediately and initiate appropriate treatment for symptoms.
- Treat overdose by maintaining airway, administering O_2, IV fluids, and give a vasopressor such as NOREPINEPHRINE.
- Treat seizures with an anticonvulsant such as PHENOBARBITAL.

OTHER REACTIONS

- Notify physician of any side effects and initiate appropriate actions.

PROCHLORPERAZINE EDISYLATE, PROCHLORPERAZINE MALEATE
Chlorazine, Compazine, Stemetil

CLASS

- Antiemetic (phenothiazine derivative)

USES

- Control of nausea and vomiting
- Management of psychotic disorders
- Used in combination with METOCLOPRAMIDE HCL for migraine headache

ACTION

Blocks chemoreceptor trigger zone and blocks vomiting center in the brain

–Antipsychotic properties appear to be related to a decrease in neural transmission in central dopamine-dependent pathways

USUAL DOSAGE/ROUTE

ADULT (nausea and vomiting)

–PO: 6–10 mg 3–4 times/day

–Rectal: 25 mg 2 times/day

–IM, IV: 5–10 mg every 3–4 hr, not to exceed 40 mg/day

ADULT (psychosis)

–PO: 5–10 mg 3–4 times/day

–IM: 10–20 mg for immediate control and repeat every 2–4 hr as needed

PEDIATRIC (nausea and vomiting, psychosis)

PO and rectal: under 2 yr or 20 lb not recommended

–20–29 lb: 2.5 mg 1–2 times/day, not to exceed 7.5 mg daily

–30–39 lb: 2.5 mg 2–3 times/day, not to exceed 10 mg daily

–40–85 lb: 2.5 mg 3 times/day or 5 mg 2 times/day, not to exceed 15 mg daily

–IM: 0.132 mg/kg; one dose usually adequate

ADVERSE/SIDE EFFECTS

RAPID

–Hypotension (immediately after injection)

–N & V

–Palpitations (immediately after injection)

–Euphoria

–Sedation

–Drowsiness

–Deep sleep

–Oculogyric crisis

–Opisthotonic posturing (especially children)

GRADUAL

–Depression

–Anorexia

–Tachycardia
–Respiratory depression

CONTRAINDICATIONS
–Hypersensitivity to drug or phenothiazines
–CNS depression
–Bone marrow depression

SPECIAL PRECAUTIONS
–Children under 2 yr
–Pregnant or lactating patients
–Elderly

OTHER SPECIAL INFORMATION
–For direct IV infusion, mix each 5 mg in 9 ml of NS and infuse over 1–2 min.
–IM injection should be given slowly and deeply.
–Oral concentrate should be diluted just before administration with at least 60 ml of water, juice, or carbonated beverage.

ANTIDOTE
SEVERE REACTIONS
–D/C drug immediately and initiate appropriate treatment for symptoms.

OTHER REACTIONS
–Notify physician of any side effects and initiate appropriate actions.

PROMETHAZINE HCL Ganphen, Methazine, Pentazine, Phenergan, Remsed, and others

CLASS
–Antihistamine (H_1-receptor antagonist)

USES

–N & V
–Symptomatic allergy relief
–Amelioration and prevention of blood and plasma reaction
–Sedation
–Adjunctive therapy with MEPERIDINE and other analgesics for pain control (has synergistic effect)

ACTION

–Acts on CNS to produce antihistaminic, sedative, amnesic, antiemetic, and antimotion sickness effects

USUAL DOSAGE/ROUTE

ADULT

–PO, Rectal, IM, IV: 12.5–50 mg repeated at 4–6 hr as needed
–*Motion sickness:* initial day, 25 mg PO 30 min to 1 hr before travel; repeated at 8–12 hr as needed; duration of travel, 25 mg on rising and at evening meal

PEDIATRIC

–PO, Rectal, IM, IV: 0.25–0.5 mg/kg or 15 mg/M^2/dose
–IV concentration not greater than 25 mg/min

ADVERSE/SIDE EFFECTS

RAPID

–Drowsiness
–Dry mouth
–Blurred vision
–Respiratory suppression
–Restlessness
–Dizziness

GRADUAL

–Constipation
–Urinary retention
–Transient hypotension
–Leukopenia
–Agranulocytosis

CONTRAINDICATIONS
–Hypersensitivity
–Acute asthma attack
–Lower respiratory tract disease
–Hypertension

SPECIAL PRECAUTIONS
–Narrow-angle glaucoma
–Stenosing peptic ulcer
–Pyloroduodenal obstruction
–Prostatic hypertrophy
–Bladder neck obstruction
–Epilepsy
–Bone marrow depression
–Severe CNS depression
–Pregnancy (except labor)
–Hepatic dysfunction
–Respiratory diseases (particularly in children)

OTHER SPECIAL INFORMATION
–Effect is potentiated by MAO inhibitors.
–Vasopressor effect of EPINEPHRINE is reversed.
–Dosage must be decreased when used concurrently with other CNS depressants.
–Irritation and necrosis may occur with extravasation or intraarterial injection.
–This drug may interfere with blood typing.
–False urine pregnancy results may occur with concurrent use.
–Inflammatory response of intradermal allergen tests may be altered.
–Monitor VS closely after administration (particularly parenteral).

ANTIDOTE

SEVERE REACTIONS
–D/C drug immediately and initiate appropriate treatment for symptoms.
–Treat PO overdose with IPECAC SYRUP or lavage.

–Treat overdose reactions with DIAZEPAM, vasopressors to lower BP and pulse, and short-acting barbiturates.

OTHER REACTIONS

Notify physician of any side effects and initiate appropriate actions.

PROPANETRIOL TRINITRATE 1–2–3 (nitroglycerin) Cardabid, Nitro-Bid, Nitrocap, Nitrocels, Nitrodisc, Nitro-Dur, Nitrol, Nitrolingual, Nitrospan, Nitrostat, Tridil, and others

CLASS

–Nitrate vasodilator

USES

–Treatment of angina pectoris
–Reduction of blood pressure
–Control of blood pressure in perioperative hypertension
–CHF associated with acute MI

ACTION

–Relaxes smooth muscle, dilation of arterial and venous beds
–Promotes peripheral pooling of blood and decreases venous return to the heart, thereby reducing systolic, diastolic, and mean arterial blood pressure

USUAL DOSAGE/ROUTE

ADULT

–SL: 0.15–0.6 mg, may repeat every 5 min for 15 min for acute attack
–Lingual spray: 0.4 mg spray, use 1–2 sprays, may repeat 3–5 min for a total of 3 sprays
–SUS CAP: one capsule every 6–12 hr on an empty stomach

–Topically: 1–2 inches every 8 hr and increase up to 4 inches as needed
–Transdermal: 1 patch/pad every day to a hair-free site
–IV: 5 mcg/min every 3–5 min, with increases by 5 mcg/min every 3–5 min until desired response (mix in 250 ml D_5W or NS)

PEDIATRIC
–Safe use in children not established

ADVERSE/SIDE EFFECTS

RAPID
–Headache
–N & V
–Flushing
–Tachycardia
–Restlessness
–Muscle twitching
–Palpitations
–Dizziness

GRADUAL
–Abdominal pain
–Postural hypotension

CONTRAINDICATIONS
–Hypersensitivity to drug or nitrites
–Severe anemia
–Increased ICP
–Cerebral hemorrhage

SPECIAL PRECAUTIONS
–Postural hypotension
–Pregnant or lactating patients

OTHER SPECIAL INFORMATION
–Nitrostat IV can react to containers, filters, and tubing; use glass bottles only; avoid using filters; use polyvinyl chloride tubing.
–Do not mix with any other drugs.

–Monitor for increased heart rate and decreased blood pressure every 5–15 min during administration.
–Tolerance to headache usually develops, but one can use non-narcotic analgesics to relieve the pain.

ANTIDOTE

SEVERE REACTIONS

–D/C drug immediately and initiate appropriate treatment for symptoms.
–Treat hypotension with vasopressors such as DOPAMINE, or METARAMINOL.

OTHER REACTIONS

–Notify physician of any side effects and initiate appropriate actions.

PROPOFOL Diprivan

CLASS

–General anesthetic (hypnotic)

USES

–Anesthesia induction and maintenance

ACTION

–Inhibits ascending pathways in the central nervous system to alter pain perception and increase pain threshold

USUAL DOSAGE/ROUTE

ADULT

–IV: induction: 2.0–2.5 mg/kg every 10 seconds until induction onset (elderly = 1.0–1.5 mg/kg every 10 seconds until induction onset)
–IV: maintenance: 0.1–0.2 mg/kg/min (elderly = 0.05–0.1 mg/kg/min)
–IV: bolus: 25–50 mg increments as needed

PEDIATRIC
–Safe use in children not established

ADVERSE/SIDE EFFECTS

RAPID
–N & V
–Abdominal cramping
–Dry mouth
–Jerking/tremor
–Shivering
–Paresthesia
–Agitation
–Eye pain
–Strong taste
–Bradycardia
–Hypotension
–ST segment depression
–Apnea
–Cough
–Hiccups
–Flushing
–Hives
–Burning/stinging at injection site
–PVCs
–PACs

GRADUAL
–Fever
–Urine retention
–Green urine
–Phlebitis

CONTRAINDICATIONS
–Hypersensitivity

SPECIAL PRECAUTIONS
–Pregnant or lactating patients
–Labor and delivery
–Respiratory depression/disorders
–Cardiac dysrhythmias

–Children
–Elderly (requires reduced dosage)

OTHER SPECIAL INFORMATION

–Onset = 40 seconds; half-life = 1–8 min; terminal half-life = 5–10 hr.
–Assess injection site for phlebitis.
–Dilute this drug with D_5W and mix only in glass containers; the drug is very unstable in plastic.

ANTIDOTE

SEVERE REACTIONS

–D/C drug immediately and initiate appropriate treatment for symptoms.
–Treat hypotension with vasopressor agents such as DOPAMINE or METARAMINOL.
–Treat overdose with anticholinergics such as ATROPINE, and ALS procedures as appropriate.

OTHER REACTIONS

–Notify physician of any side effects and initiate appropriate actions.

PROPRANOLOL HCL Inderal

CLASS

–Beta-1 (cardiac) and beta-2 (pulmonary) adrenergic blocker (antihypertensive, antianginal)

USES

–Mild-to-moderate hypertension
–Dysrhythmias
–Angina
–Migraine headache
–Postmyocardial infarction
–Pheochromocytoma

ACTION
–Acts as a beta-adrenergic receptor blocking agent

USUAL DOSAGE/ROUTE

ADULT
–*Hypertension:* PO: 100–480 mg/day in 2–3 divided doses; maximum 640 mg/day
–*Angina pectoris:* PO: 10–20 mg 3–4 times daily
–*Dysrhythmias:* PO: 10–30 mg 3–4 times daily
–*Pheochromocytoma:* PO: 30–60 mg daily in 2–4 divided doses
–IV: 0.5–3.0 mg at rate of no more than 1 mg/min; may repeat in 2 min

PEDIATRIC
–Safe use in children not established

ADVERSE/SIDE EFFECTS

RAPID
–Bronchospasm
–Dyspnea
–Bradycardia
–Hypotension
–Dry mouth
–Laryngospasm

GRADUAL
–NVD
–Mental depression
–Skin rash
–Paresthesia of hands
–Fever
–CHF
–Nightmares

CONTRAINDICATIONS
–Hypersensitivity
–Bronchial asthma
–Sinus bradycardia
–Greater than first-degree heart block

–Cardiogenic shock
–Bronchospastic disease
–Right ventricular failure secondary to pulmonary hypertension
–Persons taking MAO inhibitors

OTHER SPECIAL INFORMATION
–Monitor ECG during IV administration (watch for bradycardia).
–Observe diabetic patients carefully for insulin shock because this drug masks signs of hypoglycemia.

ANTIDOTE
SEVERE REACTIONS
–D/C drug immediately and initiate appropriate treatment for symptoms.
–Treat hypotension and circulatory collapse with ATROPINE SULFATE 0.25–1.0 mg IV.

OTHER REACTIONS
–Notify physician of any side effects and initiate appropriate actions.

PROTAMINE SULFATE Protamine Sulfate

CLASS
–Heparin antagonist

USES
–Antidote for heparin overdose

ACTION
–Alone has anticoagulant effect
–Is a strong base combining with HEPARIN (strongly acidic) to form a stable salt, neutralizing the effect of both drugs

USUAL DOSAGE/ROUTE

ADULT AND PEDIATRIC

–Slow IV: 1.0–1.5 mg per 100 units of HEPARIN given push over 1–3 min, not to exceed 50 mg within a 10-min period

ADVERSE/SIDE EFFECTS

RAPID

–Hypotension
–Bradycardia
–Dyspnea
–Anaphylaxis
–Bleeding postcardiopulmonary bypass or in persons undergoing extracorporeal dialysis

GRADUAL

–Transitory flushing
–Transitory feeling of warmth
–Hypotension
–Bradycardia
–N & V
–Rash
–Back pain
–Hemorrhage

CONTRAINDICATIONS

–Hypersensitivity to drug or to fish
–Hemorrhage not secondary to HEPARIN overdose
–Cardiovascular disease

SPECIAL PRECAUTIONS

–Pregnant or lactating patients
–Vasectomized males
–Children

OTHER SPECIAL INFORMATION

–Each milligram neutralizes approximately 90 USP units of HEPARIN in lung tissue or approximately 115 USP units of HEPARIN from intestinal mucosa.
–Onset of neutralization within 5 min; duration is approximately 2 hr.

–Dosage should be titrated by coagulation studies and time of HEPARIN dosage.
–Because this drug may be inactivated by blood, additional doses may be required if HEPARIN rebound occurs.
–Excessive administration will result in anticoagulation with subsequent hemorrhage; therefore, doses greater than 100 mg are not recommended in a short period of time.

ANTIDOTE

SEVERE REACTIONS
–D/C drug immediately and initiate appropriate treatment for symptoms.

OTHER REACTIONS
–Notify physician of any side effects and initiate appropriate actions.

QUINIDINE GLUCONATE, QUINIDINE POLYGALACTURONATE, QUINIDINE SULFATE Cardioquin, Cin-Quin, Duraquin, Quinaglute, Quinidex, and others

CLASS

–Antidysrhythmic

USES

–To treat atrial fibrillation, atrial flutter, paroxysmal atrial and supraventricular tachycardia, paroxysmal ventricular tachycardia not associated with complete heart block, premature atrial and ventricular extrasystoles
–Maintenance therapy after electrical conversion of atrial fibrillation and/or flutter

ACTION

–Acts at cellular level to depress myocardial excitability, contractility, automaticity, and conduction velocity; prolongs effective refractory period
–Blocks vagal AV node stimulation (anticholinergic action) leading to increased ventricular rate, particularly at high doses
–Produces hypotension by peripheral vasodilation and partially by alpha-adrenergic blockage

USUAL DOSAGE/ROUTE

ADULT

QUINIDINE SULFATE (dosage highly individualized)
–*Test dose:* PO: 200 mg
–PO: 10–20 mg/kg/day in 4–6 divided doses, titrate dosage to plasma concentration of 2–6 mcg/ml
–*Premature atrial and ventricular contractions:* PO: 200–300 mg 3–4 times daily
–*Paroxysmal tachycardia:* PO: 400 mg every 2–3 hr until termination of paroxysm

–*Atrial flutter:* should be preceded by digitalization, dosage highly individualized

–*Atrial fibrillation:* PO: 300–400 mg every 6 hr; if successful conversion does not occur with plasma levels of 9 mcg/ml, increased dosage leads only to side effects

–*Maintenance:* PO: 200–300 mg 3–4 times daily in 4 divided doses

–Extended action tablet: PO: 300 mg every 8–12 hr

QUINIDINE GLUCONATE (dosage highly individualized)

–*Prophylactic and maintenance therapy:* PO: 1–2 extended release tablets every 8–12 hr (each tablet = 324 mg QUINIDINE GLUCONATE)

–*Acute tachycardia:* IM: 600 mg initially; 400 mg may be repeated every 2 hr as needed (titrated to patient's response)

–IV (not preferred, use with extreme caution): 250–750 mg at a rate no greater than 1 ml (16 mg) per min

PEDIATRIC

QUINIDINE SULFATE

–*Test dose:* PO: 2 mg/kg

–*Therapeutic dose:* PO: 6 mg/kg 5 times daily

QUINIDINE GLUCONATE

–*Test dose:* PO, IM, IV: 2 mg/kg (60 mg/M^2)

–*Therapeutic dose:* PO, IM, IV: 30 mg/kg/24 hr (900 mg/M^2/24 hr) divided into 5 doses

ADVERSE/SIDE EFFECTS

RAPID

–Dizziness
–Vertigo
–Light-headedness
–Respiratory depression
–Dyspnea
–Asthma
–Hypotension
–Bradycardia
–Heart block
–Cardiac standstill

–Tremor
–Bitter taste in mouth
–Pruritus
–Urticaria

GRADUAL
–Headache
–Nausea
–Fever
–Ringing in the ears
–Confusion
–Restlessness
–Apprehension
–Diarrhea
–Visual impairment
–Hepatotoxicity
–Thrombocytopenia
–CHF
–Polyarthralgia
–Acute hemolytic anemia
–Hypoprothrombinemia
–Leukopenia

CONTRAINDICATIONS
–Hypersensitivity
–Thrombocytopenic purpura associated with prior use
–Intraventricular conduction defects
–Digitalis intoxication
–Potassium imbalance
–Thyrotoxicosis
–Acute rheumatic fever
–Subacute bacterial endocarditis
–COPD

SPECIAL PRECAUTIONS
–Pregnant or lactating patients
–Children
–Renal disease
–Liver disease
–CHF

–Respiratory depression
–Myasthenia gravis
–Hypotension

OTHER SPECIAL INFORMATION

–Discontinue if side effects increase, QRS width increases greater than 25% of original, QT interval prolongation, disappearance of P waves, sudden onset or increase in PVCs.
–Extended-release form is only for prophylactic and maintenance therapy.
–Administer with food to decrease GI irritation.
–Monitor ECG and blood pressure.
–DIGITALIS should precede QUINIDINE in treatment of atrial flutter to prevent ventricular tachycardia.
–Effect potentiated by hyperkalemia and decreased by hypokalemia.
–Strict I & O, serum electrolytes, acid/base balance monitoring necessary if diarrhea occurs.
–Embolization may occur following conversion to sinus rhythm for long-term atrial fibrillation.
–Long-term therapy requires serial renal and liver function tests and serum electrolytes and blood count testing.
–This drug may falsely increase urinary catecholamines and interfere with urinary steroid values.
–This drug potentiates effect of oral anticoagulants, anticholinergics, neuromuscular blocking agents, and DIGITALIS.
–Concurrent use of ACETAZOLAMIDE, BICARBONATE, and other urine alkalinizing agents may increase QUINIDINE plasma levels.
–Concurrent use of PHENOBARBITAL or PHENYTOIN may significantly decrease serum half-life of this drug.
–This drug cross-reacts in patients who have demonstrated QUINIDINE-induced thrombocytopenia.

ANTIDOTE

SEVERE REACTIONS

–D/C drug immediately and initiate appropriate treatment for symptoms.

–Treat overdose with OXYGEN, respiratory assistance, ALS protocols as appropriate.
–Treat circulatory depression with DOPAMINE.
–Treat convulsions with DIAZEPAM HCL or THIOPENTAL.

OTHER REACTIONS

–Notify physician of any side effects and initiate appropriate actions.

[illegible] Quinidine

RANITIDINE HCL Zantac

CLASS
–Histamine H_2-receptor antagonist

USES
–Hypersecretory conditions such as Zollinger–Ellison syndrome
–Treatment and prevention of gastric and duodenal ulcers
–Management of gastroesophageal reflux

ACTION
–Inhibits the action of histamine at the H_2-receptor site located primarily in gastric parietal cells, inhibiting gastric acid secretion

USUAL DOSAGE/ROUTE

ADULT (Zollinger-Ellison syndrome)
–PO: 150 mg 2 times daily up to 6g/day in severe disease
–IM, IV: 50 mg every 6–8 hr

ADULT (ulcer disease)
–PO: 150 mg 2 times daily or 300 mg at bedtime; preventative = 150 mg at bedtime
–IM, IV: 50 mg every 6–8 hr (up to 400 mg/day)
–*(Management of gastroesophageal reflux)* PO: 150 mg 2 times per day

PEDIATRIC
–Use in children not established

ADVERSE/SIDE EFFECTS

RAPID
–Anaphylaxis
–Dizziness
–Headache
–Malaise
–Premature ventricular contractions
–Rashes (IV)

–Nausea
–Blurred vision

GRADUAL
–Gynecomastia
–Hepatotoxicity
–Rashes (PO)
–Impotence
–Hallucination
–Blood count changes

CONTRAINDICATIONS
–Hypersensitivity

SPECIAL PRECAUTIONS
–Pregnant or lactating patients
–Elderly
–Renal impairment
–Hepatic impairment (increased risk of confusion, dosage reduction recommended)
–Children less than 12 yr (safety not established)

OTHER SPECIAL INFORMATION
–Administer with meals for prolonged drug effects.
–Space antacids one hr before or one hr after taking this drug.
–Administer IV slowly, bradycardia may occur, give over 30 min.
–This drug is metabolized by the liver, excreted in urine and breast milk.
–Instruct patient to avoid black pepper, caffeine, alcohol, harsh spices, and extremes in temperature of food
–Assess patient routinely for epigastric or abdominal pain and frank or occult blood in stool, emesis, or gastric aspirate.
–This drug may cause false-negative results for urine protein.
–Inform patient that smoking interferes with the action of this drug.
–Therapy should be continued for at least 6 weeks after initial episode.

ANTIDOTE

SEVERE REACTIONS

–D/C drug immediately and initiate appropriate treatment for symptoms.

OTHER REACTIONS

–Notify physician of any side effects and initiate appropriate actions.

SODIUM BICARBONATE Baking Soda, Bell-ans, Citrocarbonate, Neut, Soda Mint, Sodium Bicarbonate ($NaHCO_3$)

CLASS
–Alkalizing agent

USES
–Acidosis (metabolic)
–Cardiac arrest
–Gastric acidity
–Reduces acidity systemically and locally as an antipruritic

ACTION
–Restores the bicarbonate ion and elevates the pH of the blood to reverse acidosis
–Orally neutralizes gastric acid to form water, sodium chloride, and carbon dioxide

USUAL DOSAGE/ROUTE

ADULT
–PO: 325 mg–2 gm 3 or 4 times/day as needed for alkalinization
–IV push: 1 mEq/kg initially; may be repeated × 1, then 0.5 mEq/kg every 10 min until pH stable (44.6 mEq per ampule IV)
–IV infusion: 2–5 mEq/kg over 4–8 hr depending on pH and CO_2 levels

PEDIATRIC
–PO: 12–120 mg/kg/day as needed for alkalinization
–IV push: 1 meq/kg initially, then 0.5 mEq/kg every 10 min until pH is stable
–IV infusion: 2–5 mEq/kg over 4–8 hr depending on pH and CO_2 levels, not to exceed 8 mEq/kg/day

ADVERSE/SIDE EFFECTS

RAPID

–Tetany
–Hyperreflexia
–Twitching
–Convulsions

GRADUAL

–Alkalosis
–Water retention
–Edema
–Weight gain
–Paralytic ileus
–Dysrhythmias from K^+ depletion

CONTRAINDICATIONS

–Hypersensitivity
–Hypertension
–Peptic ulcer
–Renal disease

SPECIAL PRECAUTIONS

–Pregnancy
–Cirrhosis
–Toxemia
–CHF

OTHER SPECIAL INFORMATION

–Use IV to combat metabolic acidosis especially in cardiac arrest.
–If blood gases are unavailable during arrest, consider using 0.5 mEq/kg until spontaneous circulation returns.
–Do not take with milk; may cause hypercalcemia, alkalosis, and possibly renal calculi.
–This drug precipitates if mixed with CALCIUM CHLORIDE.
–IV infusion may cause extravasation and tissue sloughing.

ANTIDOTE

SEVERE REACTIONS

–D/C drug immediately and initiate appropriate treatment for symptoms.

OTHER REACTIONS
–Notify physician of any side effects and initiate appropriate actions.

STREPTOKINASE Kabikinase, Streptase

CLASS
–Thrombolytic enzyme

USES
–Coronary thrombosis associated with acute transmural MI
–Recent, severe, or massive deep vein thrombosis
–Pulmonary emboli
–Arterial embolism
–Management of occluded arteriovenous cannulae

ACTION
–Directly converts plasminogen to plasmin (fibrindysin) which subsequently dissolves fibrin deposits, including those required for normal hemostasis

USUAL DOSAGE/ROUTE
ADULT
–*Myocardial infarction (acute transmural):* IV: 1,500,000 IU–give within one hour of MI
–*Intracoronary:* IV: 20,000 IU bolus, followed by 2,000 IU/min infusion over 1 hr
–*Deep vein thrombosis, pulmonary emboli, arterial embolism, or thromboses:* IV: 250,000 IU loading dose over ½ hr followed by 100,000 IU/hr for 24 hr for pulmonary emboli, 72 hr for recurrent pulmonary emboli or deep vein thrombosis
–*Arteriovenous cannulae occlusion:* IV: 250,000 IU/2ml solution into occluded limb of cannula run over ½ hr, clamp for 2 hr, aspirate contents, flush with NaCl solution and reconnect

PEDIATRIC
–Safe use in children not established

ADVERSE/SIDE EFFECTS

RAPID
–Bleeding
–Decreased hematocrit
–Rash
–Urticaria
–Headache
–Fever
–Nausea
–Bronchospasm
–Anaphylaxis
–Periorbital edema
–Hypertension
–Shortness of breath
–Low back pain

GRADUAL
–Phlebitis at IV infusion site

CONTRAINDICATIONS
–Hypersensitivity
–Active internal bleeding
–Recent (less than 2 months) cerebrovascular accident
–Intracranial or intraspinal surgery
–Thoracic surgery
–Uncontrolled severe hypertension
–Renal disease
–Hepatic disease

SPECIAL PRECAUTIONS
–Pregnant or lactating patients
–Arterial emboli from left side of heart
–Children
–Diabetic hemorrhagic retinopathy
–Recent streptococcal infection
–Recent STREPTOKINASE therapy

OTHER SPECIAL INFORMATION
–Monitor ECG continuously.
–Cardiac enzymes should be monitored.
–Monitor pulse, blood pressure, hemodynamics, and respiratory status.
–Observe extremities and palpate pulses of affected extremities.
–Provide pressure for 30 sec to minor bleeding sites.
–Follow administration of this drug with HEPARIN infusion to increase the PTT to 1.5–2.0 × baseline for 3–7 days.

ANTIDOTE

SEVERE REACTIONS
–D/C drug immediately and initiate appropriate treatment for symptoms.
–Treat reactions with AMINOCAPROIC ACID (Amicar) for antidote
–Treat bleeding with cryoprecipitate or fresh frozen plasma

OTHER REACTIONS
–Notify physician of any side effects and initiate appropriate actions.

SUCCINYLCHOLINE CHLORIDE Anectine, Brevidil-M, Quelicin, Scoline, Sucostrin, Suxamethonium, Sux-Cert

CLASS
–Neuromuscular blockers (depolarizing-ultra short)

USES
–Anesthesia maintenance by skeletal muscle paralysis
–Skeletal muscle relaxation during mechanical ventilation
–Facilitation of endotracheal intubation
–Facilitation of orthopedic manipulations

ACTION

–Inhibits transmission of nerve impulses by binding with cholinergic receptor sites to block the effect of acetylcholine at the myoneural junction

USUAL DOSAGE/ROUTE

ADULT

–IV: Test dose: 10 mg (0.1 mg/kg), then assess respiratory function
–IV: Brief procedures: 0.6 mg/kg initially, then assess response
–IV: Prolonged procedures: 2.5 mg/min or 0.6 mg/kg initially, then 0.04–0.07 mg/kg as needed
–IM: 2.5–4.0 mg/kg not to exceed 150 mg

PEDIATRIC

–IV: Brief procedures: 1–2 mg/kg initially, then assess response
–IM: 1–2 mg/kg not to exceed 150 mg

ADVERSE/SIDE EFFECTS

RAPID

–Bradycardia
–Hypotension
–Sinus arrest
–Dysrhythmias
–Bronchospasm
–Cyanosis
–Respiratory depression
–Prolonged apnea
–Rash
–Flushing
–Pruritis
–Urticaria

GRADUAL

–Increased secretions
–Increased intraocular pressure
–Weakness
–Prolonged relaxation

–Myoglobulinemia
–Hyperkalemia

CONTRAINDICATIONS
–Hypersensitivity
–Malignant hyperthermia
–Decreased plasma pseudocholinesterase

SPECIAL PRECAUTIONS
–Pregnant or lactating patients
–Cardiac disease
–Severe burns
–Fractures
–Electrolyte imbalances (may increase action of drug)
–Dehydration
–Neuromuscular disease
–Respiratory disease
–Collagen disease
–Glaucoma/eye surgery/eye wounds
–Elderly
–Children less than 2 yr (increases risk of malignant hyperthermia)

OTHER SPECIAL INFORMATION
–IV onset = 1 min; peak = 1–3 min; duration = 4–10 min.
–IM onset = 2–3 min; duration = 10–30 min.
–Do not mix with barbiturates in solution or syringe.
–Assess neuromuscular blockade with a nerve stimulator.
–Give IV drug slowly over 1–2 minutes.
–Give IM deep into the gluteal or high deltoid muscle.
–This drug has no effect on consciousness or the pain threshold and should always include use of anesthesia or analygesics when surgical or painful procedures are performed.

ANTIDOTE
SEVERE REACTIONS
–D/C drug immediately and initiate appropriate treatment for symptoms.

–Treat overdose with an anticholinesterase (cholinergic) such as EDROPHONIUM CHLORIDE, NEOSTIGMINE, or ATROPINE, and initiate ALS procedures as required.

OTHER REACTIONS

–Notify physician of any side effects and initiate appropriate actions.

TERBUTALINE SULFATE Brethaire, Brethine, Bricanyl

CLASS

–Beta-2 (pulmonary) adrenergic agent (catecholamine)

USES

–Bronchodilator in asthma
–Reversible bronchospasm occurring with bronchitis and emphysema
–Premature labor

ACTION

–Relaxes and dilates the smooth muscle of the bronchioles

USUAL DOSAGE/ROUTE

ADULT AND PEDIATRIC (over 12 yr)

–PO: 2.5–5.0 mg 3–4 times/day not exceeding 15 mg/24 hr
–SC: 0.25–0.5 mg; may repeat × 1
–INH: 2 puffs 1 min apart, then every 4–6 hr

ADVERSE/SIDE EFFECTS

RAPID

–Tachycardia
–Palpitations
–Nervousness
–Tremor
–Anxiety
–N & V

–Dizziness
–Hypertension

GRADUAL
–Hyperglycemia
–Insomnia
–Headache

CONTRAINDICATIONS
–Hypersensitivity
–Narrow-angle glaucoma
–Tachydysrhythmias
–Angina pectoris

SPECIAL PRECAUTIONS
–Pregnancy
–Cardiac disorders
–Hyperthyroidism
–Diabetes mellitus
–Prostatic hypertrophy
–Seizure disorders

OTHER SPECIAL INFORMATION
–This drug is not recommended in children under 12 years.
–Concurrent use with PROPRANOLOL will antagonize the effects of this drug.
–Concurrent use with MAO inhibitors is contraindicated.

ANTIDOTE

SEVERE REACTIONS
–D/C drug immediately and initiate appropriate treatment for symptoms.
–Treat hypertension with alpha-blockers such as PRAZOSIN or HYTRIN.
–Treat hypotension with NOREPINEPHRINE.

TETANUS IMMUNE GLOBULIN (HUMAN)
HomoTet, Hyper-Tet, Pro-Tet, TIG

CLASS
–Tetanus vaccine plasma from immunized humans

USES
–Provides passive immunity to tetanus in patients with tetanus-prone injuries with questionable immunity

ACTION
–Provides protective levels of antibodies in the circulation for 3–4 weeks, which is the incubation period for most cases of tetanus
–Immunity is longer than with tetanus antitoxin

USUAL DOSAGE/ROUTE
ADULT AND PEDIATRIC
–IM: 250–500 units prophylactically; doses of 400–500 units may be required for high-risk situations

ADVERSE/SIDE EFFECTS
RAPID
–Pain at injection site

GRADUAL
–Low-grade fever
–Erythema

CONTRAINDICATIONS
–Hypersensitivity to drug or THIMEROSAL disinfectant

SPECIAL PRECAUTIONS
–None specified

OTHER SPECIAL INFORMATION
–Passive immunization should not be substituted for active immunization with tetanus toxoid.
–Use different injection site for each dose.

ANTIDOTE

SEVERE REACTIONS

–D/C drug immediately and initiate appropriate treatment for symptoms.

OTHER REACTIONS

–Notify physician of any side effects and initiate appropriate actions.

TETANUS TOXOID, ABSORBED, USP
Tetanus, Tetanus Toxoid

CLASS

–Toxoid (biological, immunizing agent)

USES

–Active immunization and protection against tetanus (toxins produced during infection with tetanus)

ACTION

–Invokes an immunologic response and subsequent protection against tetanus toxin

USUAL DOSAGE/ROUTE

ADULT AND PEDIATRIC

–SC, IM: 0.5 ml dose × 2 at 3-week intervals, then 0.5 ml 1 year after the second dose
–Booster recommended every 10 yr

ADVERSE/SIDE EFFECTS

RAPID

–Anaphylaxis
–N & V
–Laryngospasm

GRADUAL

–Slight fever
–Chills

–Malaise
–Aches
–Pains
–Pruritus
–Erythema
–Induration
–Nodule at site of injection
–Anorexia

CONTRAINDICATIONS

–Hypersensitivity
–Immunosuppression and immunoglobulin abnormalities
–Active tetanus infection
–Poliomyelitis

SPECIAL PRECAUTIONS

–Pregnancy

OTHER SPECIAL INFORMATION

–Obtain allergy history.
–Determine date of last tetanus immunization.
–Refrigerate toxoids.
–TETANUS TOXOID, ABSORBED is a sterile suspension precipitated or absorbed by the addition of alum, aluminum hydroxide, or aluminum phosphate to a formal dehydrated solution of the products of growth of Clostridium tetani.
–Tetanus also is available with additives for exposure to diphtheria (DT) and pertussis (DPT).

ANTIDOTE

SEVERE REACTIONS

–D/C drug immediately and initiate appropriate treatment for symptoms.
–Treat laryngospasm with EPINEPHRINE 1:1000 solution.
–Treat anaphylaxis with ALS protocols as appropriate.

OTHER REACTIONS

–Notify physician of any side effects and initiate appropriate actions.

TETRACYCLINE HCL, TETRACYCLINE PHOSPHATE COMPLEX Acromycin, Panmycin, Tetracap, Tetracyn, Tetralan, Trexin, and many others

CLASS
–Tetracycline antibiotic (broad-spectrum)

USES
–Broad-spectrum antimicrobial effective against a variety of gram-positive and gram-negative bacteria, certain mycoplasmas, rickettsiae, protozoa

ACTION
–Bacteriostatic agent that exerts its effect by blocking the attachment of aminoacyl transfer RNA to ribosomes, thus interfering with protein synthesis

USUAL DOSAGE/ROUTE

ADULT
–PO: 250–500 mg every 6 hr
–IM: 250 mg/day or 150 mg every 12 hr
–IV: 250–500 mg every 8–12 hr

PEDIATRIC (over 8 yr)
–PO: 25–50 mg/kg/day in 3–4 divided doses
–IM: 15–25 mg/kg/day in 3–4 divided doses
–IV: 10–20 mg/kg/day in 2 divided doses

ADVERSE/SIDE EFFECTS

RAPID
–NVD
–Headache
–Paresthesia
–Rash
–Urticaria

GRADUAL

–Photosensitivity
–Epigastric burning
–Maculopapular rash
–Glossitis
–Abdominal cramps
–Increased BUN
–Stomatitis
–Brown tongue
–Tooth discoloration
–Superinfection
–Increased pigmentation

CONTRAINDICATIONS

–Hypersensitivity
–Children less than 8 yr
–Pregnancy
–Lactation
–During tooth development (last trimester of pregnancy, neonatal period, and early childhood)

SPECIAL PRECAUTIONS

–Renal disease
–Liver disease

OTHER SPECIAL INFORMATION

–Renal injury (Fanconi-like syndrome) has been attributed to administration of outdated drug.
–This drug may exacerbate systemic lupus erythematosus.
–This drug decomposes with age, exposure to light, and when improperly stored.
–This drug may cause yellow–brown discoloration of teeth.
–Administer oral preparation to patient with an empty stomach to enhance absorption.
–Foods or drugs high in iron, aluminum, or calcium, such as milk and antacids, impede absorption.
–Give deep IM and no more than 2 ml in one injection site.
–Serum half-life = 6–12 hr.

ANTIDOTE

SEVERE REACTIONS

–D/C drug immediately and initiate appropriate treatment for symptoms.

OTHER REACTIONS

–Notify physician of any side effects and initiate appropriate actions.

THIAMINE HCL, USP Apatate, Betalins, Revitonus, Thia, Vitamin B_1

CLASS

–Vitamin B_1 (water-soluble)

USES

–Anemia secondary to THIAMINE deficiency
–Treatment of beriberi
GI disturbances
–Visual phenomena
–Polyneuritis secondary to alcoholism

ACTION

–Functions as an essential coenzyme in carbohydrate metabolism
–Has a role in conversion of tryptophan to nicotinamide

USUAL DOSAGE/ROUTE

ADULT

–PO: 100 mg/day
–IM: 10–500 mg/day in 2–3 divided doses
–IV: 100–500 mg single dose

PEDIATRIC

–PO: 10–50 mg/day in 2–3 divided doses
–IM: 10–50 mg/day

ADVERSE/SIDE EFFECTS

RAPID

–Anaphylactic shock (rare)
–Hypotension after rapid IV infusion
–Tightness of throat

GRADUAL

–Weakness
–Restlessness
–Pulmonary edema

CONTRAINDICATIONS

–Hypersensitivity to THIAMINE products

SPECIAL PRECAUTIONS

–Pregnancy

OTHER SPECIAL INFORMATION

–Draw THIAMINE levels throughout treatment.
–Do not mix with alkaline solutions (unstable).
–Include foods high in THIAMINE after drug therapy (i.e., liver, whole or enriched grains, legumes, yeast, beef).

ANTIDOTE

SEVERE REACTIONS

–D/C drug immediately and initiate appropriate treatment for symptoms.

OTHER REACTIONS

–Notify physician of any side effects and initiate appropriate actions.

TIMOLOL MALEATE Timoptic, Blocadren

CLASS

–Beta-adrenergic blocker (antihypertensive)

USES

–Mild-to-moderate hypertension
–Sinus tachycardia
–Tachydysrhythmias
–Angina pectoris
–Open-angle and secondary glaucoma
–Ocular hypertension

ACTION

–Blocks stimulation of beta-adrenergic receptors within vascular smooth muscles, decreasing rate of SA node discharge, heart rate, and oxygen consumption

USUAL DOSAGE/ROUTE

ADULT

–*Hypertension and MI:* PO: 10 mg 2 times/day not to exceed 60 mg/day
–*Glaucoma:* Ophthalmic: 1 drop of a 0.25–0.50% solution 2 times/day in each eye; further increases in dosage are ineffectual

PEDIATRIC

–PO, IM: Not for use in children
–*Glaucoma:* Ophthalmic: 1 drop of 0.25–0.5% solution 2 times/day in each eye

ADVERSE/SIDE EFFECTS

RAPID

–Hypotension
–Bradycardia
–NVD
–Dyspnea

GRADUAL

–CHF
–Ocular irritation (occasionally)
–Insomnia
–Dizziness
–Slight increase in resting heart rate
–Abdominal pain

–Joint pain
–Muscle pain
–Visual changes (diplopia)
–Hypoglycemia

CONTRAINDICATIONS

–Hypersensitivity
–Second- and third-degree heart block
–Sinus bradycardia
–CHF
–Cardiac failure

SPECIAL PRECAUTIONS

–Major surgery
–Pregnant or lactating patients
–Diabetes mellitus
–Renal disease
–Thyroid disease
–COPD
–Heart failure
–CAD
–Bronchospasm

OTHER SPECIAL INFORMATION

–Potentiation is possible with systemically administered beta-adrenergic blocking agents.
–Onset = 30 min; peak = 1–2 hr; duration = 24 hr.
–This drug does not reduce pupil size or visual acuity.
–This drug does not cause night blindness.
–Teach patient to apply finger lightly on lacrimal sac of eye for 1 min following administration.
–Emphasize need for regular intraocular measurements, because ocular hypertension may recur and/or progress without overt signs or symptoms.

ANTIDOTE

SEVERE REACTIONS

–D/C drug immediately and initiate appropriate treatment for symptoms.

–Treat bradycardia with IV ATROPINE SULFATE.
–Treat bronchospasm with THEOPHYLLINE.
–Treat cardiac failure with DIGITALIS, OXYGEN, diuretic, hemodialysis, and treat hypotension with a vasopressor such as NOREPINEPHRINE.

OTHER REACTIONS

–Notify physician of any side effects and initiate appropriate actions.

TISSUE-TYPE PLASMINOGEN ACTIVATOR (rt-PA) Activase, Alteplase

CLASS

–Thrombolytic (tissue plasminogen activator)

USES

–Acute management of myocardial infarction, within 4–6 hr of onset of chest pain

ACTION

–Binds to fibrin to stimulate conversion of plasminogen in thrombi to plasmin
–Limits infarct size by lysis of thrombi

USUAL DOSAGE/ROUTE

ADULT

–IV (more than 65 kg): Total 100 mg over 3 hr; 60 mg over 1 hour (6–10 mg IV bolus in first 1–2 min, then remainder); 20 mg over 2nd hr, 20 mg over 3rd hr
–IV (less than 65 kg): 1.25 mg/kg total dose over 3 hr; 0.75 mg/kg over 1st hr (0.075–1.25 mg/kg IV bolus over 1st 1–2 min then remainder); 0.25 mg/kg over 2nd hr, 0.25 mg/kg over the 3rd hr

PEDIATRIC

–Safe use in children not established

ADVERSE/SIDE EFFECTS

RAPID

–Dysrhythmias
–Bleeding (GI, retroperitoneal, intracranial)
–Surface bleeding
–Bradycardia
–Headache
–Epistaxis
–N & V
–Musculoskeletal pain
–Fever
–Rash

GRADUAL

–Phlebitis at IV infusion site

CONTRAINDICATIONS

–Hypersensitivity
–Active bleeding
–Within 2 months of cranial or spinal surgery
–Intracranial neoplasm
–Severe hypertension
–Arteriovenous malformation
–Known bleeding tendencies
–Recent trauma

SPECIAL PRECAUTIONS

–Pregnant or lactating patients
–Within 10 days of major surgery, trauma, GI or GU bleeding
–Cerebrovascular disease
–Uncontrolled hypertension
–Severe liver disease
–Severe renal disease
–Persons more than 75 yr old
–Within first 10 postpartum days
–In conjunction with oral anticoagulant therapy
–Children

OTHER SPECIAL INFORMATION

- Initially monitor vital signs every 15 min; notify physician for systolic greater than 180 mmHg or diastolic greater than 110 mmHg.
- Monitor ECG continuously.
- Monitor heart and breath sounds; notify physician of signs of congestive heart failure, S_3, jugular vein distension.
- Monitor for signs of bleeding—stools, puncture sites, epistaxis, ecchymosis.
- Monitor Hct, platelets, PTT, PT, TT, APTT.
- Begin HEPARIN therapy after thrombolytic therapy is discontinued.
- This drug must be given within 6 hr of coronary occlusion for best results.

ANTIDOTE

SEVERE REACTIONS

- D/C drug immediately and initiate appropriate treatment for symptoms.
- Treat reactions with AMINOCAPROIC ACID.
- Treat bleeding with fresh frozen plasma or cryoprecipitate.

OTHER REACTIONS

- Notify physician of any side effects and initiate appropriate actions.

TOLAZAMIDE Ronase, Tolamide, Tolinase

CLASS

- Antidiabetic (first generation oral hypoglycemic sulfonylurea)

USES

- Treatment for stable or adult onset diabetes (type II) which cannot be controlled by diet alone

ACTION

–Decreases serum glucose by stimulation of pancreatic beta cells to synthesize and reduce insulin; also increases active insulin receptor sites

USUAL DOSAGE/ROUTE

ADULT

–Individually adjusted PO: 100–250 mg daily, up to 1000 mg/day; if more than 500 mg is required, it should be given 2 times/day

PEDIATRIC

–Not for use in children

ADVERSE/SIDE EFFECTS

RAPID

–Hypoglycemia
–Dizziness
–Headache
–Weakness
–Vertigo

GRADUAL

–Bone marrow aplasia
–Fatigue
–NVD
–Aplastic anemia
–Hyponatremia
–Photosensitivity

CONTRAINDICATIONS

–Hypersensitivity to drug or sulfa drugs
–Juvenile diabetes (type I)
–Severe trauma
–Severe renal disease
–Impending surgery
–Severe liver disease
–Severe endocrine diseases
–Ketosis, acidosis, coma
–Alcoholism

SPECIAL PRECAUTIONS
–Severe cardiovascular disease
–Elderly (dosage reduction required)
–Infection
–Severe stress
–Pregnancy

OTHER SPECIAL INFORMATION
–No action occurs if functional beta cells are not present.
–Observe patient for S & S of hypoglycemia (sweating, hunger, weakness, dizziness, tremor, tachycardia, anxiety).
–Administer once-a-day dose 30 min before breakfast to ensure best diabetic control.
–Tablets may be crushed and taken with fluids if patient has difficulty swallowing.
–Urine checks for glucose and ketones essential before meds and at bedtime.

ANTIDOTE

SEVERE REACTIONS

–D/C drug immediately and initiate appropriate treatment for symptoms.
–Treat hypoglycemia with oral glucose or with $D_{50}W$ followed by a continuous IV infusion of a dilute dextrose ($D_{2½}W$) to keep blood sugar levels at approximately 100 mg/dl.

OTHER REACTIONS

–Notify physician of any side effects and initiate appropriate actions.

TOLBUTAMIDE, TOLBUTAMIDE SODIUM
Mobenol, Novobutamide, Oramide, Orinase, Tollutone

CLASS
–Antidiabetic (first-generation oral hypoglycemic sulfonylurea)

USES
–Treatment for stable or adult onset diabetes (type II) which cannot be controlled by diet alone
–Adjunctive therapy in stabilization of certain cases of insulin-dependent, maturity-onset diabetes mellitus
–Diagnostic agent to rule out islet cell tumor

ACTION
–Decreases serum glucose by stimulation of pancreatic beta cells to synthesize and release insulin; also increases active insulin receptor sites

USUAL DOSAGE/ROUTE
ADULT
–PO: initially 1–2 gm/day; adjusted per patient's response for minimal effective dosage in the range of 0.25–3.0 gm; maintenance dose greater than 3 gm/day seldom necessary; total dose may be taken in the morning; preferred in divided doses before meals
–IV (diagnostic, TOLBUTAMIDE SODIUM): 1 gm in sterile water over 2–3 min

PEDIATRIC
–Not for use in children

ADVERSE/SIDE EFFECTS
RAPID
–Hypoglycemia
–Dizziness
–Headache
–Weakness
–Vertigo

GRADUAL
–Fatigue
–Aplastic anemia
–Hyponatremia
–Photosensitivity
–NVD
–Bone marrow aplasia

–Rash
–Urticaria
–Thrombocytopenia
–Leukopenia
–Agranulocytosis
–Pancytopenia
–Cholestatic jaundice

CONTRAINDICATIONS
–Hypersensitivity to drug or sulfa drugs
–Juvenile diabetes (type I)
–Severe stress
–Severe infection
–Severe trauma
–History of acidosis or coma
–Renal disease
–Liver disease
–Thyroid, pituitary, or adrenal dysfunction
–Before and during surgery
–Fever
–Cardiac failure
–Alcoholism

SPECIAL PRECAUTIONS
–Pregnancy
–Elderly (dosage reduction required)
–Infection
–Severe stress
–Severe cardiovascular disease

OTHER SPECIAL INFORMATION
–No action occurs if functional beta cells are not present.
–Onset of oral action = 30 min; peak = 3–5 hr; half-life = 5 hr; duration = 6–12 hr.
–This drug alters liver function tests.
–This drug should not be taken at bedtime.
–Early hypoglycemia can be corrected by eating soluble glucose such as fruit juice, LifeSavers, soft drinks.
–Urine checks for glucose and ketones are essential before meals and at bedtime.

–Weight should be monitored at least once a week; a continuing weight gain necessitates discontinuation of drug.
–Concurrent use of MAO inhibitors, oral anticoagulants, salicylates, alcohol, sulfonamides, insulin, phenylbutazone, oxyphenbutazone, and chloramphenicol will enhance hypoglycemia.
–Response is decreased with concurrent use of thiazide diuretics and glucocorticosteroids.

ANTIDOTE

SEVERE REACTIONS
–D/C drug immediately and initiate appropriate treatment for symptoms.
–Treat hypoglycemia with oral glucose or with $D_{50}W$ followed by a continuous IV infusion of a dilute dextrose ($D_{2\frac{1}{2}}W$) to keep blood sugar levels at approximately 100 mg/dl.

OTHER REACTIONS
–Notify physician of any side effects and initiate appropriate actions.

TRIMETHAPHAN CAMSYLATE Arfonad

CLASS
–Antihypertensive (ganglionic blocker)

USES
–Rapid reduction of blood pressure in hypertensive emergencies
–Controlled hypotension during surgery and in clients with acute aortic dissection

ACTION
–Blocks nerve transmission at both sympathetic and autonomic ganglia to produce vasodilation

USUAL DOSAGE/ROUTE

ADULT

–IV infusion: Dilute 500 mg in 500 ml of D_5W and run at 1–5 mg/min beginning with 0.5 mg/min and increasing to maintain BP at desired range

PEDIATRIC

–IV infusion: 50–150 mcg/kg/min beginning with the smallest dose and increasing to maintain BP at desired range

ADVERSE/SIDE EFFECTS

RAPID

–Respiratory arrest
–Apnea
–NVD
–Dry mouth
–Headache
–Agitation
–Restlessness
–Rash
–Urticaria
–Pruritus
–Pupillary dilation
–Hypotension

GRADUAL

–Anorexia
–Constipation
–Weakness
–Blurred vision
–Diplopia
–Urinary retention

CONTRAINDICATIONS

–Hypersensitivity
–Uncorrected respiratory insufficiency
–Pregnant or lactating patients
–Hypovolemic shock
–Glaucoma
–Uncorrected anemia
–Anemia

SPECIAL PRECAUTIONS
–Elderly
–Debilitatetd
–Cardiac disease
–Degenerative CNS disease
–Liver disease
–Renal disease
–Diabetes mellitus
–Addison's disease
–Children

OTHER SPECIAL INFORMATION
–IV infusion onset = 1–2 min; duration = 15–30 min.
–Diuretics increase the effect of this drug.
–Do not mix with any other drug.
–Perform daily weights and I & O while on this drug
–Monitor BP and heart rhythm frequently while on this drug.

ANTIDOTE

SEVERE REACTIONS
–D/C drug immediately and initiate appropriate tretment for symptoms.
–For hypotension, administer vasopressor such as DOPAMINE or METARAMINOL.

OTHER REACTIONS
–Notify physician of any side effects and initiate appropriate actions.

TRIMETHOBENZAMIDE HCL Spengan, Ticon, Tigan

CLASS
–Antiemetic (anticholinergic)

USE
–Control of nausea and vomiting

ACTION
–Blocks the chemoreceptor trigger zone in the medulla, which acts on the vomiting center

USUAL DOSAGE/ROUTE

ADULT
–PO: 250 mg 3 or 4 times daily
–Rectal: 200 mg 3 or 4 times daily
–IM: 200 mg 3 or 4 times daily

PEDIATRIC
–PO: 100 mg 3 or 4 times daily
–Rectal: 100 mg 3 or 4 times daily
–IM: Not for use in children

ADVERSE/SIDE EFFECTS

RAPID
–Drowsiness
–Blurred vision
–Dry mouth
–Hypotension
–Convulsions
–Headache
–Rash
–Urticaria
–Coma (Reye's syndrome)

GRADUAL
–Blood dyscrasias
–Jaundice
–Insomnia
–Anorexia

CONTRAINDICATIONS
–Hypersensitivity to drug or narcotics
–In children with viral illness; may contribute to Reye's syndrome
–Shock

SPECIAL PRECAUTIONS
–Children
–Elderly
–Cardiac dysrhythmias
–Pregnancy
–Asthma
–Prostatic hypertrophy
–Glaucoma
–Peptic ulcer
–Pyloric stenosis

OTHER SPECIAL INFORMATION
–Administer deep IM into gluteus of adults.
–Avoid alcohol and other CNS depressants.

ANTIDOTE

SEVERE REACTIONS
–D/C drug immediately and initiate appropriate tretment for symptoms.

OTHER REACTIONS
–Notify physician of any side effects and initiate appropriate actions.

TRIMETHOPRIM, CO-TRIMOXAZOLE, SULFAMETHOXAZOLE Apo-Sulfatrim, Azo-Gantanol, Bactrim, Bethaprim, Co-Trim, Comoxol, Septra, Sulfatrim

CLASS
–Antibiotic (antimicrobial sulfomamide)

USES
–Urinary tract infections, especially acute and chronic cystitis
–Pneumocystic carinii
–Chancroid

–Escherichia coli
–Klebsiella
–Hemophilus influenzas
–Proteus mirabilis
–Some streptococci
–Shigellosis

ACTION

–Blocks 2 consecutive steps in bacterial synthesis of essential nucleic acids and protein

USUAL DOSAGE/ROUTE

ADULT

–PO: 160 mg TRIMETHOPRIM and 800 mg SULFA every 12 hr for 10–14 days

PEDIATRIC

–PO: 8 mg/kg TRIMETHOPRIM and 40 mg/kg SULFA per 24 hr in 2 divided doses every 12 hr (10 days for urinary tract infection; 5 days in shigellosis)

ADVERSE/SIDE EFFECTS

RAPID

–Anaphylaxis
–NVD
–Abdominal pain
–Convulsions

GRADUAL

–Stevens–Johnson syndrome
–Dermatitis
–Hepatitis
–Headache
–Insomnia
–Depression
–Aseptic meningitis
–Leukopenia
–Thrombocytopenia
–Renal failure
–Increased BUN and creatinine

CONTRAINDICATIONS
–Hypersensitivity
–Pregnancy at term
–Lactation
–Infants less than 2 months
–Folate deficiency
–G6PD deficiency
–Bronchial asthma
–Porphyria

SPECIAL PRECAUTIONS
–Severe renal impairment (dosage reduction required)
–Pregnant or lactating patients
–Renal disease
–Elderly
–Liver disease

OTHER SPECIAL INFORMATION
–Drink a full glass of water with each dose.
–Report skin rash, fever, or sore throat.
–Take 1 hr before or 2 hr after meals for best absorption.

ANTIDOTE
SEVERE REACTIONS
–D/C drug immediately and initiate appropriate treatment for symptoms.

OTHER REACTIONS
–Notify physician of any side effects and initiate appropriate actions.

TUBERCULIN PURIFIED PROTEIN DERIVATIVE (PPD) Aplisol, Mantoux, PPD, Tubersol

CLASS
–In vivo diagnostic (Mantoux)

USES

–Diagnostic screening for sensitivity to products of the tubercle bacillus resulting from previous infection

ACTION

–Injection of aqueous solution of purified protein derivative isolated from culture filtrate of human-type stain of Mycobacterium tuberculosis produces a local inflammatory reaction at injection site in person previously infected with tubercle bacillus (T.B.)

USUAL DOSAGE/ROUTE

ADULT AND PEDIATRIC

–*Usual dose* ID: 5 TU (of 5 TU/0.1 ml solution)

–*Highly sensitive person* ID: 1 TU (of 1 TU/0.1 ml solution)

–*Persons who fail to react to 1 TU or STU* ID: 250 TU (of 250 TU/0.1 ml solution)

ADVERSE/SIDE EFFECTS

RAPID

–Anaphylaxis

–Urticaria

–Edema

GRADUAL

–Pruritus

–Ulceration

CONTRAINDICATIONS

–Hypersensitivity

–Previous allergic reaction

–Previously documented tuberculosis

SPECIAL PRECAUTIONS

–History of allergies

OTHER SPECIAL INFORMATION

–Test should be administered with a disposable syringe using a 26- or 27-gauge, ½-inch needle inserted bevel up into the most superficial skin layer; a definite white bleb about

6–10 mm in diameter will appear at the needle point and will disappear within min.
–Test should be repeated at least 5 cm from original site if inadvertently delivered SC.
–Preferred site is the flexor or dorsal surface of the forearm approximately 4 inches below the elbow bend.

INTERPRETATION

–Read 48–72 hr after administration; only induration should be considered in interpretation, measured at widest distinctly palpable diameter.
–Positive reaction: palpable induration of 10 mm or more
–Doubtful: induration of 5–9 mm; retesting other forearm at higher concentration indicated; in case of known contact, should be interpreted as positive
–Negative: induration less than 5 mm
–Erythema of less than 10 mm is not significant; erythema greater than 10 mm and absence of induration may be secondary to too deep injection; retesting indicated.
–Chest X-ray should be used for persons with positive PPD reaction to determine presence or absence of pulmonary tuberculosis.
–250 TU test dose is never to be used for initial injection.
–Concurrent use of corticosteroid or immunosuppressive agents; concurrent/recent immunization with certain virus vaccines (measles, influenza) or presence of viral infection (such as rubeola, influenza, mumps) may suppress/depress reactivity to test up to 4–6 weeks.

ANTIDOTE

SEVERE REACTIONS

–D/C drug immediately and initiate appropriate treatment for symptoms.

OTHER REACTIONS

–Notify physician of any side effects and initiate appropriate actions.

UROKINASE Abbokinase, Win-Kinase

CLASS
–Thrombolytic enzyme (beta-hemolytic streptococcus filtrate)

USES
–Lysis of coronary artery emboli after MI
–Treatment of pulmonary emboli
–Management of occluded IV catheter

ACTION
–Activates plasminogen to change to plasmin which promotes thrombolysis

USUAL DOSAGE/ROUTE
ADULT
–*Pulmonary emboli:* IV: 4400 IU/kg/hr × 12–24 hr; maximum dose 200 ml followed by HEPARIN.
–*Coronary artery occlusion:* IV: 2500–10,000 U of HEPARIN bolus IV then 6000 IU/min up to 2 hr
PEDIATRIC
–Safe use in children not established

ADVERSE/SIDE EFFECTS
RAPID
–Hypertension
–Nausea
–Anaphylaxis
–Bleeding
–Shortness of breath
–Bronchospasm
–Rash
–Fever
–Headache
–Periorbital edema
GRADUAL
–Low back pain

CONTRAINDICATIONS

–Hypersensitivity
–Active bleeding
–CNS neoplasm
–Severe hypertension
–Renal or hepatic disease
–CVA within last 2 months
–Recent cranial or spinal surgery

SPECIAL PRECAUTIONS

–Pregnant or lactating patients
–Trauma or surgery within last 2 months
–Cerebrovascular disease
–Diabetic hemorrhagic retinopathy
–Arterial emboli from left side of heart
–Children

OTHER SPECIAL INFORMATION

–Monitor vital signs and bleeding every 15 min first hr, every 15–30 min during next 8 hr, and every 4 hr for duration of therapy.
–For pulmonary emboli and coronary thrombosis, monitor ECG continuously.
–Monitor Hct, Hgb, platelet count, PT, TT, APTT.

ANTIDOTE

SEVERE REACTIONS

–D/C drug immediately and initiate appropriate treatment for symptoms.
–Treat anaphylaxis with EPINEPHRINE, AMINOPHYLLINE, O_2, IV corticosteroids, antihistamines, and ALS procedures as appropriate.
–For bleeding, infuse whole blood, packed red blood cells, fresh frozen plasma, cryoprecipitate.
–Treat reactions with AMINOCAPROIC ACID (Amicar).

OTHER REACTIONS

–Notify physician of any side effects and initiate appropriate actions.

VASOPRESSIN Pitressin

CLASS
–Pituitary hormone (antidiuretic)

USES
–Treatment of central diabetes insipidus due to deficient antidiuretic hormone
–Management of abdominal distention postoperatively
–Treat bleeding esophogeal varices
–Used to eliminate gas shadows during abdominal X rays

ACTION
–Alters the permeability of the renal collecting ducts, allowing reabsorption of water
–Causes vasoconstriction in large doses

USUAL DOSAGE/ROUTE
ADULTS
–*Central diabetes insipidus:* IM, SC: 5–10 units 2–4 times/day as needed (aqueous VASOPRESSIN); 2.5–5.0 units every 2–3 days (VASOPRESSIN TANNATE)
–*Abdominal distention:* IM: 5 units initially, may increase to 10 units if necessary (aqueous)
–*GI bleeding:* IV: 0.2–0.4 units/min (aqueous), may be increased up to 0.9 units/min
–Intraarterial: 0.1–0.5 units/min
–*Preparation for GI X rays:* IM, SC: 10 units at 2 hr and again at 30 min prior to X rays

PEDIATRIC
–*Central diabetes insipidus:* IM, SC: 2.5–10 units of VASOPRESSIN 3–4 times daily, or 1.25–2.5 units every 1–3 days (VASOPRESSIN TANNATE)

ADVERSE/SIDE EFFECTS
RAPID
–Dizziness
–"Pounding" sensation in head

–Chest pain
–MI
–Abdominal cramps
–N & V
–Sweating
–Water intoxication
–Allergic reaction

GRADUAL
–Perioral blanching
–Rhinitis

CONTRAINDICATIONS
–Hypersensitivity to this drug, beef/pork proteins, or peanut oil
–Chronic renal failure with increased BUN
–Chronic nephritis

SPECIAL PRECAUTIONS
–Pregnant or lactating patients
–Comatose patients
–Seizures
–Migraine headaches
–Asthma
–Heart failure
–Elderly patients
–Children
–Renal impairment
–Coronary artery disease

OTHER SPECIAL INFORMATION
–Monitor ECG periodically throughout therapy.
–Assess patient for signs/symptoms of dehydration.
–Weigh patient daily.
–Monitor intake and output.
–Assess for edema.
–Monitor urine specific gravity throughout therapy.

ANTIDOTE

SEVERE REACTIONS

–D/C drug immediately and initiate appropriate treatment for symptoms.

–Treat overdose with MANNITOL, hypertonic DEXTROSE, UREA, and/or FUROSEMIDE.

–Maintain water restriction until polyuria returns.

OTHER REACTIONS

–Notify physician of any side effects and initiate appropriate actions.

VERAPAMIL HCL Calan, Calan SR, Cordilox, Isoptin, Isoptin SR, Veradil

CLASS

–Calcium antagonist (slow-channel blocker)

USES

–Angina pectoris

–Supraventricular tachydysrhythmias

–Hypertension

ACTION

–Blocks entry of extracellular calcium into cardiovascular cells, decreasing myocardial contractility and oxygen demand, and dilating coronary arteries and arterioles

USUAL DOSAGE/ROUTE

ADULT

–PO: 80–160 mg 3–4 times/day

–PO, SR: 240 mg SR tablet once daily in the morning

–IV: 0.075–0.15 mg/kg (5–10 mg) over 2–3 min; may repeat in 30 min

PEDIATRIC

–IV bolus (1–15 yr): 0.1–0.3 mg/kg (2–5 mg) over 2 min; may repeat in 30 min (Use in children is controversial.)

–IV bolus (0–1 yr): 0.1–0.2 mg/kg (0.75–2.0 mg) over 2 min; may repeat in 30 min (Use in infants is controversial.)

ADVERSE/SIDE EFFECTS

RAPID

–Dizziness
–Peripheral edema
–Bradycardia
–Tremors
–Dizziness
–Headache
–Dysrhythmias

GRADUAL

–Heart block
–Transient hypotension
–CHF
–Ventricular asystole
–Constipation
–Nausea
–Elevated liver enzymes
–Edema
–Fatigue

CONTRAINDICATIONS

–Hypersensitivity
–Severe hypotension
–Cardiogenic shock
–Second- or third-degree AV block
–Wolff–Parkinson–White Syndrome
–Severe CHF
–Patients on digitalis glycosides (may cause toxicity)

SPECIAL PRECAUTIONS

–Elderly
–Children
–MI
–Sick sinus syndrome
–CHF
–Liver disease

–Renal disease
–Patients on beta-blockers (may cause heart failure)

OTHER SPECIAL INFORMATION

–Do not use if patient is near digitalis toxicity.
–Give under continuous ECG monitoring.
–Give all IV infusions slowly over at least 3 min to minimize the risk of adverse reactions.

ANTIDOTE

SEVERE REACTIONS

–D/C drug immediately and initiate appropriate treatment for symptoms.
–Treat AV block with ATROPINE SULFATE, CALCIUM CHLORIDE.
–Treat hypotension with vasopressor such as DOPAMINE or METARAMINOL.

OTHER REACTIONS

–Notify physician of any side effects and initiate appropriate actions.

WARFARIN SODIUM Carfin, Coumadin, Panwarfin, Sofarin, Warfilone Sodium, Warnerin

CLASS
–Anticoagulant

USES
–Myocardial infarction
–Adjunct in coronary occlusion
–Atrial fibrillation with embolization
–Prophylaxis and treatment of pulmonary and venous thrombosis
–Pulmonary emboli

ACTION
–Inhibits precoagulation factor synthesis (factors II, VII, IX, X) in the liver by antagonizing the action of vitamin K

USUAL DOSAGE/ROUTE
ADULT
–PO: 10–15 mg/day for 3–5 days until desired prothrombin time; then adjust dosage according to day of therapeutic prothrombin time response
Example: day 1 maintenance dose 2 mg; day 2 maintenance dose 2.5–5.0 mg; day 3 maintenance dose 5.0–7.5 mg; day 4 maintenance dose 7.5–10 mg

PEDIATRIC
–Safe use in children not established

ADVERSE/SIDE EFFECTS
RAPID
–Diarrhea
–Rash
–Fever

GRADUAL
–May color the urine orange
–N & V

–Hemorrhage from any tissue or organ
–Anorexia
–Hepatitis

CONTRAINDICATIONS
–Hypersensitivity
–Hemophilia
–Leukemia with bleeding
–Peptic ulcer disease
–Thrombocytopenia purpura
–Pregnancy
–Blood dyscrasias
–Severe liver disease
–Severe hypertension
–Recent or impending surgery
–Subacute bacterial endocarditis
–Acute nephritis

SPECIAL PRECAUTIONS
–Alcoholism
–Elderly

OTHER SPECIAL INFORMATION
–Drugs that potentiate WARFARIN SODIUM include salicylates, CHLORAL HYDRATE, CLOFIBRATE, DISULFIRAM, PHENYLBUTAZONE, METHYLPHENIDATE, and sulfonamides.
–Drugs that decrease the effect of WARFARIN SODIUM include barbiturates, ETHCHLORVYNOL, GLUTETHIMIDE, and GRISEOFULVIN.
–This drug potentiates PHENYTOIN and TOLBUTAMIDE.
–Usual desired prothrombin time is 2–2½ times normal with COUMADIN therapy.
–Some patients may require extremely high doses (200 mg).
–Administer drug at the same time each day to maintain steady blood levels.
–Avoid all invasive procedures that may cause bleeding during therapy.

ANTIDOTE

SEVERE REACTIONS

–D/C drug immediately and initiate appropriate treatment for symptoms.

–With prothrombin time greater than 2½ normal administer fresh frozen plasma and/or vitamin K.

–Antidote is PHYTONADIONE (Vitamin K).

OTHER REACTIONS

–Notify physician of any side effects and initiate appropriate actions.

Part Four
Conversion Formulas and Tables

Volume Equivalents

Metric	Apothecary	Household
1 ml	15 minims	15 gtts
4 ml	1 dram	1 scant teaspoon
5 ml	1¼ drams	1 teaspoon (60–75 gtts)
15 ml	4 fluid drams (½ ounce)	1 tablespoon (3 teaspoons)
30 ml	1 fluid ounce	2 tablespoons
250 ml (¼ liter)	8 fluid ounces	1 cup (240 ml)
375 ml	12 fluid ounces	—
500 ml (½ liter)	1 pint	16 ounces (480 ml)
1000 ml (1 liter)	1 quart	32 ounces
4000 ml (4 liters)	1 gallon	128 ounces

Weight Equivalents

Metric	Apothecary
0.4 mg	1/150 grain
0.5 mg	1/120 grain
0.6 mg	1/100 gram
1 mg (0.001 gram or 1000 micrograms)	1/60 grain
60 mg (0.06 gram)	1 grain
1000 mg (1 gram)	15 grains
4 grams	60 grains (1 dram)
28.35 grams	480 grains (1 ounce)
454 grams	1.33 pounds
0.37–0.375 kilograms	1 pound
1000 grams (1 kilogram)	2.2 pounds

Formula for Medication Dosage Calculation

$$\frac{\text{Dosage available}}{\text{Dose required}} \times \frac{\text{How supplied}}{\text{Units to be administered}}$$

Example:

Give 20 mg of a drug that comes 15 mg per ml.

$$\frac{\text{Dose available is 15 mg}}{\text{Dose required is 20 mg}} \times \frac{\text{How supplied is 1 ml}}{\text{Units to be administered is } X \text{ ml}}$$

$$\frac{15 \text{ mg}}{20 \text{ mg}} \times \frac{1 \text{ ml}}{X \text{ ml}}$$

Cross multiply

$$15X = 20$$

$$X \text{ ml} = \frac{20}{15} = 1.25 \text{ ml}$$

Formulas for Intravenous Flow Rate Calculation

$$\frac{\text{Total volume to be infused}}{\text{Total time for infusion in min}} \times \text{Drop factor of tubing in drops/ml} = \text{drops/min}$$

Example:

To infuse 1000 ml of D_5W over 8 hr, what would be the drops per minute using 15 gtt/ml tubing?

$$\frac{\text{Total volume to be infused is 1000 ml}}{\text{Total time for infusion is 480 min}} \times \text{Drop factor of tubing in drops/ml is 15}$$

$$\frac{1000\text{ ml}}{480\text{ min}} \times 15 = \frac{15{,}000}{480} = 31.2 \text{ or } 31 \text{ gtts/min}$$

Hint: If you know ml/hr, the gtts/min are as follows:

Drop factor of tubing		*Drops per min*	*Using example of 100 ml/hr*
60 gtts/cc (microdrip)	=	Same as ml/hr infusing	100 gtts/min
20 gtts/cc	=	⅓ of ml/hr infusing	33 gtts/min
15 gtts/cc	=	¼ of ml/hr infusing	25 gtts/min
12 gtts/cc	=	⅕ of ml/hr infusing	20 gtts/min
10 gtts/cc	=	⅙ of ml/hr infusing	17 gtts/min

Formulas for Pediatric Dosages Calculation

Clark's Rule: Based on body weight only; should be used for children over age 2; the younger the child, the less accurate the dosage

$$\frac{\text{Child's weight (lb)} \times \text{Average adult dose}}{150 \text{ lbs}} = \text{Child's dose}$$

Example: 75-lb child using 500 mg of a drug

$$\frac{75 \text{ lbs} \times 500 \text{ mg}}{150 \text{ lbs}} = \frac{37{,}500}{150} = 250 \text{ mg}$$

Fried's Rule: Based on age only; should be used to verify dosages for children under age 1

$$\frac{\text{Child's age (months)} \times \text{Average adult dose}}{150 \text{ months}} = \text{Child's dose}$$

Example: a 9-month child using 500 mg of a drug

$$\frac{9 \text{ mos} \times 500 \text{ mg}}{150 \text{ months}} = \frac{4{,}500}{150} = 30 \text{ mg}$$

Young's Rule: Based on age only; should be used for children aged 2–12 years

$$\frac{\text{Child's age (yr)} \times \text{Average adult dose}}{\text{Child's age (yr)} + 12} = \text{Child's dose}$$

Example: a 4-yr-old child using 500 mg of a drug

$$\frac{4 \text{ yr} \times 500 \text{ mg}}{4 \text{ yr} + 12} = \frac{2000}{16} = 125 \text{ mg}$$

Formulas for Approximate Weights (kg) of Children

Age	Weight Formula (kg)	Example
3–12 months	$\frac{\text{Age (mo)} + 9}{2}$	$\frac{6 \text{ mos} + 9}{2} = \frac{15}{2} = 7.5$ kg
1–6 years	Age (yr) $\times 2 + 8$	4 yrs $\times 2 + 8 = 16$ kg
6.1–12 years	$\frac{\text{Age (yr)} \times 7 - 5}{2}$	$\frac{8 \text{ yrs} \times 7 - 5}{2} = \frac{51}{2} = 25.5$ kg

Table of Approximate Weights (kg) of Children

Age	Approx. Weight (kg)
Newborn	3
3 mos	6
6 mos	7.5
9 mos	9
12 mos (1 yr)	10
18 mos (1½ yr)	11
24 mos (2 yr)	12
30 mos (2½ yr)	13
36 mos (3 yr)	14
3½ yr	15
4 yr	16
4½ yr	17
5 yr	18
5½ yr	19
6 yr	20
6½ yr	20.25
7 yr	22
7½ yr	23.75
8 yr	25.5
8½ yr	27.25
9 yr	29
9½ yr	30.75
10 yr	32.5
10½ yr	34.25
11 yr	36
11½ yr	37.75
12 yr	39.5

Pounds-to-Kilograms Conversion Table
(2.2 lb = 1 kg)

Pounds	Kilograms	Pounds	Kilograms
0.5	0.023	66	30
1	0.455	......	......
1.5	0.682	77	35
2	0.9091	88	40
2.2	1	99	45
4.4	2	110	50
6.6	3	121	55
8.8	4	132	60
11	5	143	65
13.2	6	154	70
15.4	7	165	75
17.6	8	176	80
19.8	9	187	85
22	10	198	90
24.2	11	209	95
26.4	12	220	100
28.6	13	231	105
30.8	14	242	110
33	15	253	115
35.2	16	264	120
37.4	17	275	125
39.6	18	286	130
41.8	19	297	135
44	20	308	140
46.2	21	319	145
48.2	22	330	150
50.6	23	341	155
52.8	24	352	160
55	25	363	165
57.2	26	374	170
59.2	27	385	175
61.6	28	396	180
63.8	29	407	185

Inches-to-Centimeters Conversion Table
(1 inch = 2.54 cm)

(Feet)	Inches	Centimeters
	1	2.54
	2	5.08
	3	7.62
	4	10.16
	5	12.70
(½ foot)	6	15.24
	7	17.78
	8	20.32
	9	22.86
	10	25.40
	11	27.94
(1 foot)	12	30.48
	13	33.02
	14	35.56
	15	38.10
	16	40.64
	17	43.18
(1½ feet)	18	45.72
	19	48.26
	20	50.80
	21	53.34
	22	55.88
	23	58.42
(2 feet)	24	60.96
	25	63.50
	26	66.04
	27	68.58
	28	71.12
	29	73.66
(2½ feet)	30	76.20
	31	78.74
	32	81.28
	33	83.82
	34	86.36

(cont'd.)

Inches-to-Centimeters Conversion Table (cont'd.)
(1 inch = 2.54 cm)

(Feet)	Inches	Centimeters
	35	88.90
(3 feet)	36	91.44
	38	96.52
	40	101.60
(3½ ft)	42	106.68
	44	111.76
	46	116.84
(4 feet)	48	121.92
	50	127.00
	52	132.08
(4½ ft)	54	137.16
	56	142.24
	58	147.32
(5 feet)	60	152.40
	62	157.48
	64	162.56
(5½ ft)	66	167.64
	68	172.72
	70	177.80
(6 feet)	72	182.88
	74	187.96
	76	193.04
(6½ ft)	78	198.12
	80	203.20
	82	208.28
(7 feet)	84	213.36
	86	218.44
	88	223.52
	90	228.60

Centigrade-to-Fahrenheit Conversion Formulas and Table

To convert Centigrade (C) to Fahrenheit (F): $\frac{9 \times C}{5} + 32 = F$

To convert Fahrenheit (F) to Centigrade (C): $(F - 32) \times \frac{5}{9} = C$

Fahrenheit Degrees	Centigrade Degrees	Fahrenheit Degrees	Centigrade Degrees
106	41.1	100.6	38.1
105.8	41	100.4	38.0
105.6	40.9	100.2	37.9
105.4	40.8	100	37.8
105.2	40.7	99.8	37.7
105	40.6	99.6	37.6
104.8	40.4	99.4	37.4
104.6	40.3	99.2	37.3
104.4	40.2	99	37.2
104.2	40.1	98.8	37.1
104	40	98.6	37.0
103.8	39.9	98.4	36.9
103.6	39.8	98.2	36.8
103.4	39.7	98	36.7
103.2	39.6	97.8	36.6
103	39.4	97.6	36.4
102.8	39.3	97.4	36.3
102.6	39.2	97.2	36.2
102.4	39.1	97	36.1
102.2	39.0	96.8	36.0
102	38.9	96.6	35.9
101.8	38.8	96.4	35.8
101.6	38.7	96.2	35.7
101.4	38.6	96	35.6
101.2	38.4	95.8	35.4
101	38.3	95.6	35.3
100.8	38.2	95.4	35.2

(cont'd.)

Centigrade-to-Fahrenheit Conversion Formulas and Table (cont'd.)

Fahrenheit Degrees	Centigrade Degrees	Fahrenheit Degrees	Centigrade Degrees
95.2	35.1	92.4	33.6
95	35.0	92.2	33.4
94.8	34.9	92	33.3
94.6	34.8	91.8	33.2
94.4	34.7	91.6	33.1
94.2	34.6	91.4	33.0
94	34.4	91.2	32.9
93.8	34.3	91	32.8
93.6	34.2	90.8	32.7
93.4	34.1	90.6	32.6
93.2	34.0	90.4	32.4
93	33.9	90.2	32.3
92.8	33.8	90	32.2
92.6	33.7		

Body Surface Area of Adults (M^2)

Note: Using a straightedge, connect the patient's height in the left-hand column to his weight in the right-hand column. The place where this line intersects with the center scale estimates the body surface area.

Reproduced from Lenter, C. (ed.), *Geigy Scientific Tables*, 8th edition. Courtesy CIBA-GEIGY, Basle, Switzerland.

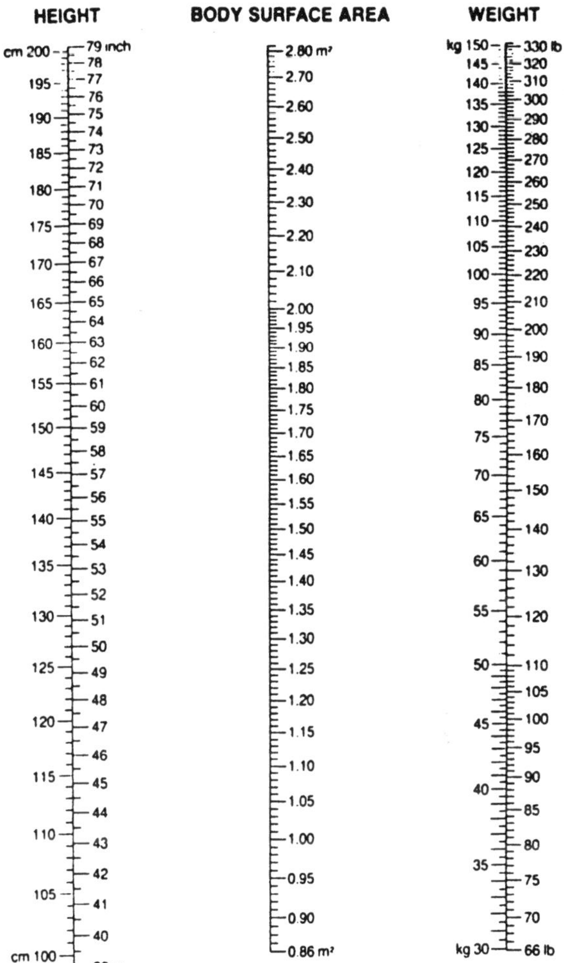
HEIGHT
BODY SURFACE AREA
WEIGHT
cm 200 – 79 inch
cm 100 – 39 in
195, 190, 185, 180, 175, 170, 165, 160, 155, 150, 145, 140, 135, 130, 125, 120, 115, 110, 105
78, 77, 76, 75, 74, 73, 72, 71, 70, 69, 68, 67, 66, 65, 64, 63, 62, 61, 60, 59, 58, 57, 56, 55, 54, 53, 52, 51, 50, 49, 48, 47, 46, 45, 44, 43, 42, 41, 40
2.80 m²
2.70, 2.60, 2.50, 2.40, 2.30, 2.20, 2.10, 2.00, 1.95, 1.90, 1.85, 1.80, 1.75, 1.70, 1.65, 1.60, 1.55, 1.50, 1.45, 1.40, 1.35, 1.30, 1.25, 1.20, 1.15, 1.10, 1.05, 1.00, 0.95, 0.90
0.86 m²
kg 150 – 330 lb
145, 140, 135, 130, 125, 120, 115, 110, 105, 100, 95, 90, 85, 80, 75, 70, 65, 60, 55, 50, 45, 40, 35
320, 310, 300, 290, 280, 270, 260, 250, 240, 230, 220, 210, 200, 190, 180, 170, 160, 150, 140, 130, 120, 110, 105, 100, 95, 90, 85, 80, 75, 70
kg 30 – 66 lb

Body Surface Area of Children (M^2)

Note: For pediatric patients of average size, body surface area may be estimated with the scale on the left. Match weight to corresponding surface area. For other pediatric patients, use the scale on the right. Place a straightedge on the correct height and weight of your patient. The place where the line connecting height and weight intersects the center scale is the surface area.

Reproduced from *Nelson Textbook of Pediatrics,* 13th edition. Courtesy W.B. Saunders Co., Philadelphia, Pa.

FOR CHILDREN OF NORMAL HEIGHT AND WEIGHT

NOMOGRAM

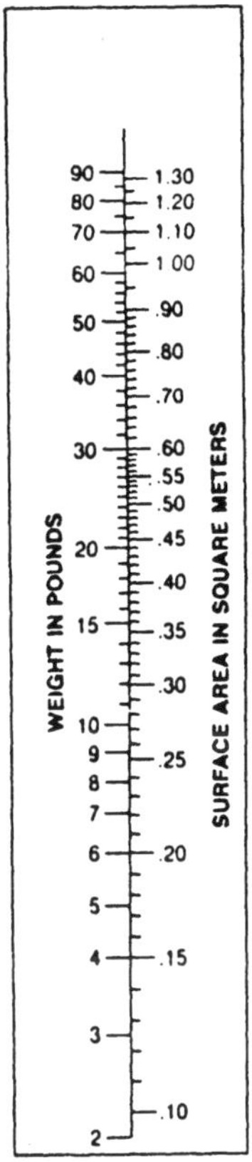

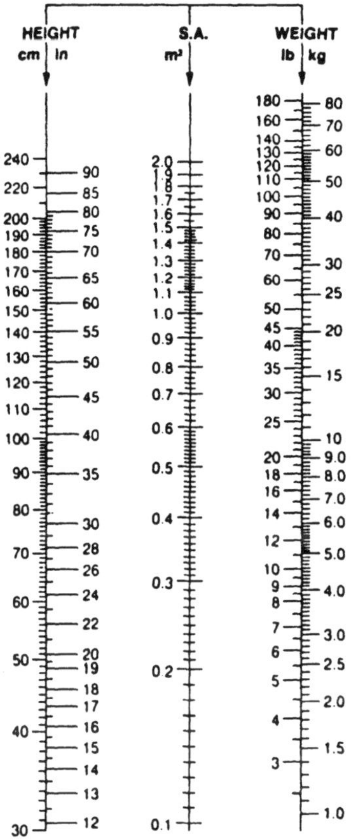

Part Five
Normal Scales, Indexes, and Scores

Adult Glasgow Coma Scale (GCS)

Physical Sign		Response	Points	Score
Eye opening		Spontaneous	4	
		To verbal stimuli	3	
		To painful stimuli	2	
		None	1	____
Best motor response (upper limb)		Obeys command	6	
	To pain	Localizes	5	
		Withdraws	4	
		Abnormal flexion*	3	
		Abnormal extension**	2	
		None	1	____
Best verbal response		Oriented	5	
		Confused	4	
		Inappropriate words	3	
		Nonspecific sounds	2	
		None	1	____
Total		Apply this score to GCS portion of Trauma Score	3–15	____

Score: (Possible 3–15, decreasing with injury severity) Total ____

*Formerly known as decorticate rigidity
**Formerly known as decerebrate rigidity

Physical Sign	Response	Points	Score

Pediatric Glasgow Coma Scale (PGCS)

Physical Sign		Response	Response	Points	Score
		<1 Year	**>1 Year**		
Eye opening		Spontaneous	Spontaneous	4	
		To shout	To verbal stimuli	3	
		To pain	To pain	2	
		None	None	1	____
		<1 Year	**>1 Year**		
Best motor response (upper limb)		Normal spontaneous movements	Obeys commands	6	
	To pain	Localizes	Localizes	5	
		Withdraws	Withdraws	4	
		Abnormal flexion*	Abnormal flexion*	3	
		Abnormal extension**	Abnormal extension**	2	
		None	None	1	____
		<2 Years	**2–5 Years**		
Best verbal response		Smiles, coos, cries appropriately	Appropriate words & phrases	5	
		Appropriate cry	Inappropriate words	4	
		Inappropriate cry or scream	Cries or screams	3	
		Grunts/moans	Grunts	2	
		None	None	1	____

Score: (Possible 3–15, decreasing with injury severity) Total ____

*Formerly known as decorticate rigidity
**Formerly known as decerebrate rigidity

Adult Prehospital Index (PHI)

Physical Sign	Value	Points	Score
Systolic BP (mmHg)	>100	0	
	86–100	1	
	75–85	2	
	<75	5	____
Pulse rate (per min)	>120	3	
	51–120	0	
	<50	5	____
Respiratory status	Normal	0	
	Labored/shallow	3	
	<10/min, needs ETT	5	____
Level of consciousness	Normal	0	
	Confused/combative	3	
	No intelligible words	5	____
Score: (Possible 0–24, increasing with injury severity; generally 0–3 = minor trauma, 4–24 = major trauma)		0–24*	Total ____

*For penetrating abdominal or chest injuries, add 4 points to the total.

Adult Trauma Score (ATS)

Parameter	Value	Points	Score
Respiratory rate (per min)	10–24	4	
	25–35	3	
	>35	2	
	<10	1	
	Apneic	0	____
Respiratory expansion (effort)	Normal	1	
	Shallow	0	
	Retractive	0	____
Systolic BP (mmHg)	>90	4	
	70–90	3	
	50–69	2	
	<50	1	
	No pulse	0	____

(cont'd.)

Adult Trauma Score (ATS) *(cont'd.)*

Parameter	Value	Points	Score
Capillary refill	Normal (<2 sec)	2	
	Delayed (>2 sec)	1	
	None	0	____
Glasgow Coma Scale	14–15	5	
	11–13	4	
	8–10	3	
	5–7	2	
	3–4	1	____
Score: (Possible 1–16, decreasing with injury severity; generally >13 = minor trauma (stable), <13 = major trauma)		Total	____

Revised Adult Trauma Score (RATS)

Parameter	Value	Points	Score
Respiratory rate (per min)	10–29	4	
	>29	3	
	6–9	2	
	1–5	1	
	0	0	____
Systolic BP (mmHg)	>89	4	
	76–89	3	
	50–75	2	
	1–49	1	
	No pulse	0	____
Glasgow Coma Scale	13–15	4	
	9–12	3	
	6–9	2	
	4–5	1	
	3	0	____

Score: (Possible 1–12, decreasing with injury severity; generally 10–12 = minor trauma (stable), <10 = trauma alert) Total ____

Pediatric Trauma Score (PTS)

	Points			
Patient Information	+2	+1	−1	Score
Weight	>44 lbs (>20 kg)	22–44 lbs (10–20 kg)	<22 lbs (<10 kg)	____
Airway	Normal & patent without assistance	(Maintainable) Oral or nasal airway; head positioning required	(Unmaintainable) Intubated; tracheostomy; invasive	____
Systolic BP (mmHg)	>90 and/or palpable radial pulse	50–90 and/or palpable femoral/carotid pulse	<50 and/or no palpable pulse	____
Level of consciousness (LOC)	Completely awake; normal mental status & LOC	Obtunded or any history of decreased LOC	Comatose; unresponsive	____
Open wound	None	Minor abrasions, contusions, lacerations	Major or penetrating, or burns	____

Fractures	None	Single closed or suspected	Open, or closed multiple	____
Score: (Possible −6 to +12, decreasing with injury severity; generally 9–12 = minor trauma, 6–8 = potentially life-threatening, 0–5 = life-threatening, <0 = usually fatal)				____

Severity of Burns Table

	Degree		
Severity	1°	2°	3°
Minor	<20%	<15%	<2%
Moderate	>20%	>15%	>2%
Severe	—	>30%	>10%

Parkland Formula for IV Fluids for the First 8 Hours

$$\frac{\%\ \text{Burn area} \times \text{pt. weight (kg)}}{4} = \text{ml/hr}$$

Example:

$$\frac{20\% \times 50\ \text{kg}}{4} = \frac{1000}{4} = 250\ \text{ml/hr for first 8 hr}$$

Adult and Pediatric Burn Charts (Rule of Nines)

Adult and Pediatric Burn Charts (Rule of Nines)

Infant

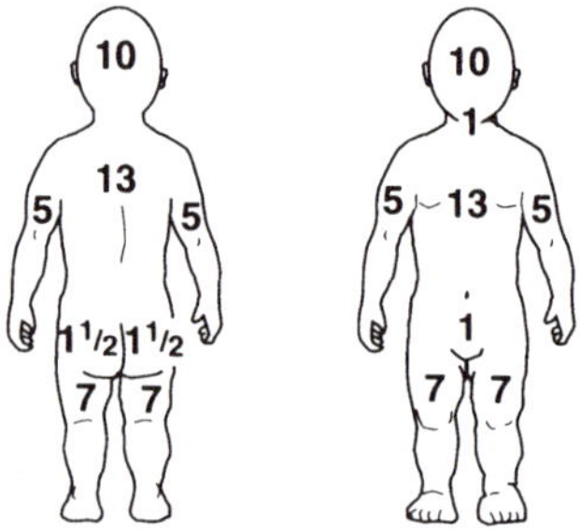

Pediatric

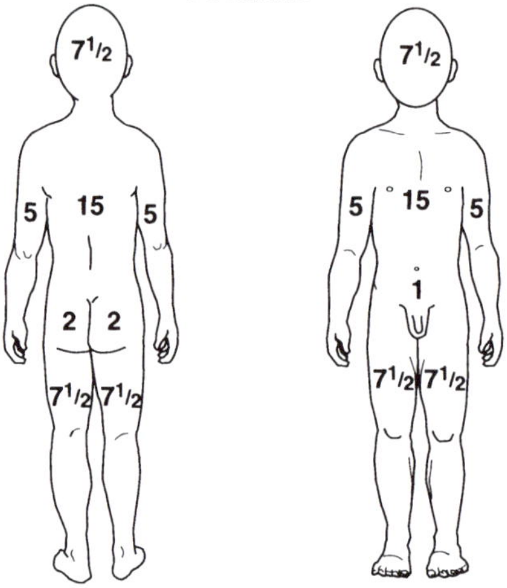

Adult

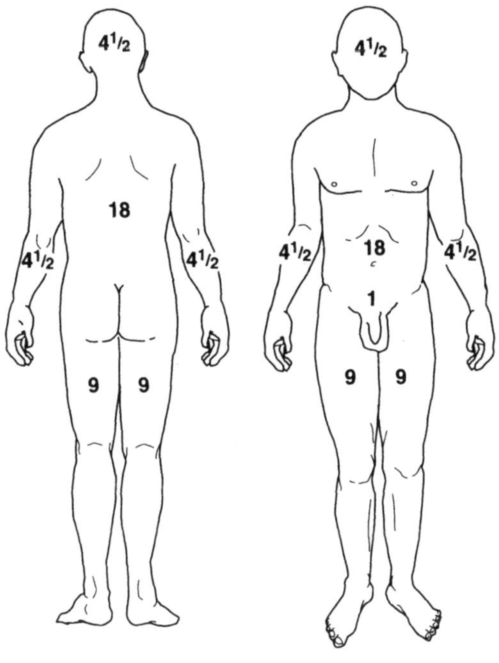

Infant Apgar Scoring Chart*

Sign	Score: 0	Score: 1	Score: 2
Appearance (Color)	Blue, pale	Pink body, blue extremities	All pink
Pulse (Heartrate)	Absent	< 100/min	> 100/min
Grimace (Reflex Irritability)	Absent	Grimace to stimulation	Cough or sneeze to stimulation
Activity (Muscle tone)	Limp	Some flexion of extremities	Active motion, full flexion
Respiration (Respiratory effort)	Absent	Slow, irregular	Robust cry

*Scoring ranges from 1–10, with 7–10 suggesting little or no deterioration from asphysia. Degree of clinical depression is scored at 1 min. and 5 mins. after birth. Deterioration occurs in a predictable manner: First color, then respiration, then tone, then reflex, and finally heart rate.

Pediatric Normal Vital Sign Parameters

Age	Mean wt in kg	Minimum Syst BP	Normal HR	Normal RR
Premature	1.0	38	120–170	40–60
Premature	2.0	40	120–170	40–60
Premature	2.5	40	120–170	40–60
Term	3.5	50	100–170	40–60
3 mo	6.0	50	100–170	30–50
6 mo	8.0	60	100–170	30–50
1 yr	10.0	65	100–170	30–40
2 yr	13.0	65	100–160	20–30
4 yr	15.0	70	80–130	20
6 yr	20.0	75	70–115	16
8 yr	25.0	80	70–110	16
10 yr	30.0	85	60–105	16
12 yr	40.0	90	60–100	16

Guide for EKG Interpretation

When examining an EKG strip, determine:

1. Rate (# R waves in a 6-second strip; or # 0.20 blocks between R–R interval divided into 300; or # 0.04 blocks between R–R interval divided into 1500).
2. Rhythm (regular or irregular) (Atrial and ventricular)
3. P wave(s) (present, absent, inverted, following QRS interval)
4. PR interval (*N* = 0.10–0.20 sec)
5. QRS interval (*N* = <0.12 sec)
6. QT interval (*N* = 0.36–0.44 sec or <½ of R—R interval)
7. Diagnosis of rhythm
8. Treatment(s) of choice (Interventions)

12-Lead EKG ruler

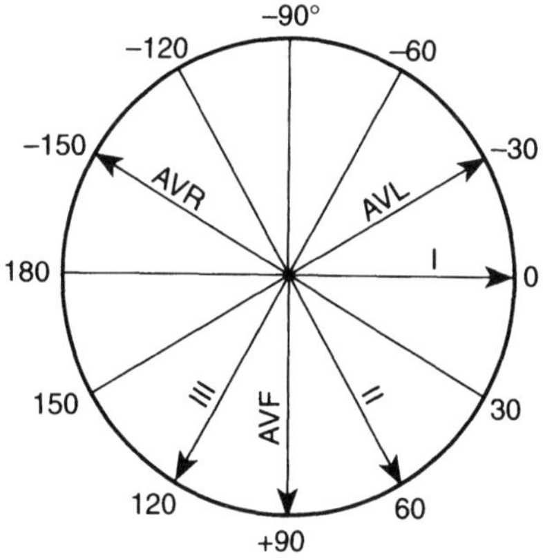

Acute MI Findings on EKG

Anterior Wall:	Q waves & ST elevation in I, AVL, V1–V4
Anterolateral:	Q waves & ST elevation in V1–V6
Apical Wall:	Q waves & ST elevation in V5–V6
Inferior Wall:	Q waves & ST elevation in II, III, & AVF
Lateral Wall:	Q waves in I, AVL V4–V6
Posterior Wall:	R waves & ST depression in V1–V2
Ventricular Septum:	Q waves & ST elevation in V1–V2

Appendix

List of Abbreviations

A.C.L.S.:	Advanced Cardiac Life Support
ALS:	Advanced Life Support
ADH:	antidiuretic hormone
AHFS:	American Hospital Formulary Service
APTT:	activated partial thromboplastin time
AV:	atrioventricular
BP:	blood pressure
BUN:	blood urea nitrogen
CA^{++}:	calcium
CaCl:	calcium chloride
CAD:	coronary artery disease
cc:	cubic centimeter(s)
CDC:	Centers for Disease Control
CHF:	congestive heart failure
Cl:	chloride
cm:	centimeter(s)
CNS:	central nervous system
CO:	carbon monoxide
CO_2:	carbon dioxide
COLD:	chronic obstructive lung disease
COPD:	chronic obstructive pulmonary disease
Cr:	creatinine
CVP:	central venous pressure
D/C:	discontinue

ECG, EKG:	electrocardiogram
EEG:	electroencephalogram
ESR:	erythrocyte sedimentation rate
ET:	endotracheal tube
GI:	gastrointestinal
gr:	grain(s)
gm, g:	gram(s)
gt, gtt:	drop(s)
GU:	genitourinary
HCL:	hydrochloride
Hct:	hematocrit
hr:	hour(s)
ICP:	intracranial pressure
ID:	intradermal
I & O:	input and output
IM:	intramuscular
IO:	intraosseous
IPPB:	intermittent positive pressure breathing
IV:	intravenous
K^+:	potassium
kg:	kilogram(s)
lb:	pound(s)
LOC:	level of consciousness
M^2:	meters squared (body surface area)
MAO:	monoamine oxidase
max:	maximum
mcg:	microgram(s)
mEq, meq:	milliequivalent(s)
mg:	milligram(s)
min:	minute(s)
ml:	milliliter(s)
mmHg:	millimeters of mercury
Na^+:	sodium
NaCl:	sodium chloride
$NaHCO_3$:	sodium bicarbonate
NF:	National Formulary
NPO:	nothing by mouth
NS:	normal saline
N & V:	nausea and vomiting

NVD:	nausea, vomiting, and diarrhea
O_2:	oxygen
PAC:	premature atrial contraction
PCO_2:	Partial pressure carbon dioxide
PE:	pulmonary edema
pH:	hydrogen–ion concentration
PO, po:	per OS (by mouth)
PO_2:	partial pressure oxygen
PPD:	purified protein derivative
PRBC:	packed red blood cells
PT:	prothrombin time
PTT:	partial thromboplastin time
PVC:	premature ventricular contraction
q.d.:	once every day
RBC:	red blood cells
S & S:	signs and symptoms
SA:	sinoatrial
SC, sc:	subcutaneous
sec:	second(s)
SGOT:	serum glutamic pyruvic transaminase
SL:	sublingual
sol:	solution
SQ:	subcutaneous
Tbsp:	tablespoon(s)
tsp:	teaspoon(s)
TU:	tuberculin unit(s)
U, u:	unit(s)
USP:	United States Pharmacopeia
VS:	vital signs
WBC:	white blood cells
wt:	weight
yr:	year(s)
<:	less than
>:	greater than

BIBLIOGRAPHY

Alfaro-LeFevve, R., Blicharz, M. E., Flynn, N. M., & Boyer, M. J. (1992). *Drug handbook: A nursing process approach.* Redwood City, CA: Addison-Wesley Publishing Company.

American Heart Association. (1990). *Textbook of advanced cardiac life support* (2nd ed.). Dallas: Author.

American Heart Association. (1990). *Textbook of pediatric advanced life support* (2nd ed.) Dallas: Author.

American Hospital Formulary Service: Drug Information 91. (1991). Bethesda, MD: American Society of Hospital Pharmacists.

Benson, D. S., & Conte, R. R. (1991). *91/92 nursing meds.* Norwalk: Appleton & Lange.

Behrman, R., Vaughan, V., & Nelson, W. (Eds.). (1987). *Nelson textbook of pediatrics.* Philadelphia: W. B. Saunders Company.

Boyer, M. J. (1987). *Math for nurses.* St. Louis: J. B. Lippincott Company.

Burrell, L. O. (1992). *Adult nursing in hospital and community settings.* Norwalk: Appleton and Lange Publishers.

Clochesy, J., Breu, C., Cardin, S., Rudy, E., & Whittaker, A. (1993). *Critical care nursing.* Philadelphia: W. B. Saunders.

Deglin, J. H., Vallerand, A. H., & Russin, M. M. (1991). *Davis's drug guide for nurses* (2nd ed.). Philadelphia: F. A. Davis Company/Publishers.

Gahart, B. L. (1992). *Intravenous medications: A handbook for nurses and other allied health personnel.* St. Louis: The C. V. Mosby Company.

Govoni, L. E., & Hayes, J. E. (1988). *Drugs and nursing implications.* Norwalk, CT: Appleton & Lange.

Grossman, M., & Dieckmann, R. A. (1991). *Pediatric emergency medicine: A Clinician's Reference.* St. Louis: J. B. Lippincott Company.

Klaus, M., & Fanaroff, A. (1986). *Care of the high-risk neonate.* Philadelphia: W. B. Saunders Company.

Kuhn, M. M. (1991). *Pharmacotherapeutics: A nursing*

process approach (2nd ed.). Philadelphia: F. A. Davis Company/Publishers.

Lee, G. (1991). *Flight nursing: Principles and practice.* St. Louis: Mosby Year Book, Inc.

Lee, G. (1992). *Quick emergency care reference.* St. Louis: Mosby Year Book, Inc.

LeSage, P., Derr, P., & Tardiff, J. (1990). *E.M.S. field guide* (6th ed.). Lake Oswego: Creative Ventures, Incorporated.

Madigan, K. G. (1990). *Prehospital emergency drugs pocket reference.* St. Louis: The C. V. Mosby Company.

McKenry, L. M., & Salerno, E. (1992). *Mosby's pharmacology in nursing* (18th ed). St. Louis: Mosby Year Book, Inc.

Merenstein, G., & Gardner, S. (1989). *Handbook of neonatal intensive care.* St. Louis: The C. V. Mosby Company.

Nentwich, P. F. (1991). *1991–1992 handbook of intravenous medications.* Boston: Jones and Bartlett Publishers.

Nursing 91 drug handbook. (1991). Springhouse, PA: Springhouse Corporation.

Olsen, J. L., Ablan, L. J., Giangrasso, A. P., & Siner-Weissmon, H. (1987). *Medical dosage calculations* (4th ed.). Reading, MA: Addison-Wesley Publishing Company.

Opie, L. H. (1987). *Drugs for the heart* (2d ed.). Orlando: Harcourt Brace Jovanovich Publications.

Phipps, W. J., Long, B. C., Woods, N. F., & Cassmeyer, V. L. (1991). *Medical-surgical nursing: Concepts and clinical practice.* St. Louis: Mosby Year Book, Inc.

Physicians' desk reference. (1991). Oradell: Litton Industries, Incorporated.

Physician's 1992 drug handbook. (1992). Springhouse, PA: Springhouse Corporation.

Sheehy, S. B. (1992). *Emergency nursing: Principles and practice* (3rd ed.). St. Louis: Mosby Year Book, Inc.

Skidmore-Roth, L. (1992). *Mosby's 1992 nursing drug reference.* St. Louis: The C. V. Mosby Company.

Springhouse Corporation. (1990). *Handbook of pediatric drug therapy.* Springhouse, PA: Author.

Suddarth, D. S. (1991). *The Lippincott manual of nursing practice* (5th ed.). New York: J. B. Lippincott Company.

Thelan, L., Davie, J., & Urden, L. (1990). *Textbook of critical care nursing: Diagnosis and management.* St. Louis: The C. V. Mosby Company.

Thompson, S. (1990). *Emergency care of children.* Boston: Jones and Bartlett Publishers.

Underhill, S. L., Woods, S. L., Froelicher, E. S. S., & Halpenny, C. J. (1990). *Cardiovascular medications for cardiac nursing.* Philadelphia: J. B. Lippincott Company.

Weinstein, S. M. (1991). *The nurses' handbook of intravenous medications.* New York: J. B. Lippincott Company.

GENERIC

TRADE

Class

Uses

Action

Usual Dosage/Route

Adult

Pediatric

Adverse/Side Effects

Rapid

Gradual

Contraindications

Special Precautions

Other Special Information

Antidote

Severe Reactions

Other Reactions

GENERIC

TRADE

Class

Uses

Action

Usual Dosage/Route

Adult

Pediatric

Adverse/Side Effects

Rapid

Gradual

Contraindications

Special Precautions

Other Special Information

Antidote

Severe Reactions

Other Reactions

Index

Generic names are in all caps; trade names are in lower case.

9 780867 202144

Printed in Dunstable, United Kingdom

91343134R00268